PROSTATE CANCER

Second Edition

A Man's Guide to Treatment

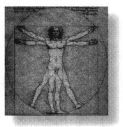

Arthur Centeno, M.D.

Addicus Books
Omaha, Nebraska

An Addicus Nonfiction Book

ISBN
Cover design by George Foster
Illustrations and typography by Jack Kusler

This book is not intended to be a substitute for a physician, nor do the authors intend to give advice contrary to that of an attending physician.

Library of Congress Cataloging-in-Publication Data

Centeno, Arthur, 1953-
  Prostate cancer : a man's guide to treatment / Arthur Centeno, M.D.—Second [edition].
     pages cm
  Includes bibliographical references and index.
  ISBN 978-1-940495-40-8 (alk. paper)
  1. Prostate—Cancer—Popular works. I. Title.
  RC280.P7C46 2014
  616.99'463—dc23

2014009643

Addicus Books, Inc.
P.O. Box 45327
Omaha, Nebraska 68145
www.AddicusBooks.com

Printed in the United States of America
10 9 8 7 6 5 4 3 2 1

To the memory of my late wife, Virginia, and to the memory of my patients who have lost their battles with cancer. They have taught me about the human spirit, the will to live, and the dignity of fighting the good fight.

Contents

Introduction

If you have been diagnosed with prostate cancer, you are not alone. Some 200,000 men are diagnosed with the disease annually in the United States. As you may already know, a diagnosis of cancer is the beginning of a journey that none of us would choose to take. It is a journey that most of us begin with fear and trepidation. But thanks to modern medicine, many of our fears can be put to rest. Much can be done to fight prostate cancer. And that fight is often won, especially when the cancer is diagnosed early.

Having treated thousands of patients, I have learned that one of the ways a patient can combat fear and anxiety is to become an active participant in his treatment. This means learning about the disease and the treatment options. The more you know, the less you face the unknown. Knowledge helps take away some of the fear.

It is my hope that this book will help you make smart decisions and take responsibility for managing prostate cancer and its treatment. No book, however complete, can substitute for your doctor's expertise and advice. But with the information on these pages and in the scores of other excellent resources for prostate cancer patients and their loved ones, you can be an active partner in the disease's management and possibly in its cure.

Prostate Cancer: An Overview

If you have been told that you have prostate cancer, your first reaction might well have been panic, numbness, despair, or a combination of these feelings. Many people experience a dizzying whirl of emotions after receiving a cancer diagnosis—anger, depression, concern for family and loved ones, fear of the unknown, and sometimes a nameless dread that comes and goes in those first days and weeks.

All this is natural and normal. You'd be less than human if you didn't grieve, at least briefly, for the loss of your "old" life.

Even so—though you might find this hard to believe right now—there are thousands and thousands of prostate cancer survivors who will tell you the diagnosis was one of the best things that ever happened to them. Once they got over the initial shock and started looking for answers and finding support, they saw life as the wonderful gift it truly is. They educated themselves about the disease and the many ways of dealing with it. They discovered that knowledge is power and learned to use that power for their own health and well-being. They forged new relationships, strengthened existing ones, and shared— perhaps for the first time—their deepest feelings and greatest fears.

Through this process, these survivors learned that prostate cancer is curable—yes, curable—when found in the early stages. And they saw how their own decisions and actions could help them stay healthy for many years to come.

The Prostate Gland

To better understand prostate cancer, let's first examine the role of the prostate gland itself. The *prostate* is a muscular gland about the size and shape of a walnut. Part of the urinary and reproductive systems, it is located in the pelvis below the urinary bladder and sits just in front of the rectum. The *urethra,* which carries urine and semen out of the body through the penis, runs through the prostate like a straw through a doughnut hole.

Because it is actually several small glands encased in the *prostate capsule,* the prostate is sometimes described as having two lobes, three lobes, or several zones. Of these, the *peripheral zone,* or outer zone, where most prostate cancer begins, is the largest; the muscular *central zone* prevents semen from backing up into the bladder during ejaculation; and the *transition zone,* which surrounds the urethra, is the only site for a common noncancerous disorder called *benign prostatic hyperplasia (BPH).*

The Prostate and Reproduction

Your prostate gland is small but mighty. It weighs between 20 and 40 grams. By comparison, a first-class letter weighs 30 grams. Small as it is, the prostate is essential for normal human reproduction. It adds important fluid and nutrients to sperm during ejaculation. Among these nutrients are citric acid, potassium, calcium, and zinc. To function properly, the prostate depends on male hormones *(androgens),* chiefly *testosterone.* Testosterone

Prostate Gland

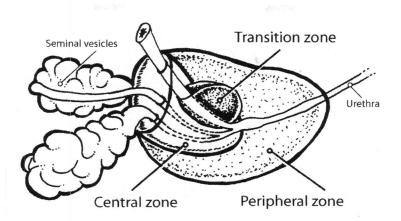

Seminal vesicles
Transition zone
Urethra
Central zone
Peripheral zone

is responsible for the traits usually associated with men—body hair, deep voice, musculature, and so on. The prostate converts testosterone to another, more potent male hormone, *dihydrotestosterone* or *DHT.*

Of course, the prostate alone does not fuel the reproductive process. The *testicles* or *testes* manufacture sperm and most of the testosterone upon which the prostate depends. The *adrenal glands* also produce small amounts of androgens. A small gland, the *epididymis,* sits next to the testes and stores sperm until they mature. Just before the male orgasm, numerous muscles work together to produce semen and pump it out of the body. These muscles squeeze *seminal fluid* from the prostate and from the adjacent seminal vesicles through small pores into the urethra, where two 12-inch tubes called *vasa deferentia* deposit sperm. The vasa deferentia and the ducts of the seminal vesicles join in the prostate to form the *ejaculatory duct.* During ejaculation, sperm and seminal fluid—the components of semen—travel through the urethra and exit the penis.

Prostate Gland Side View

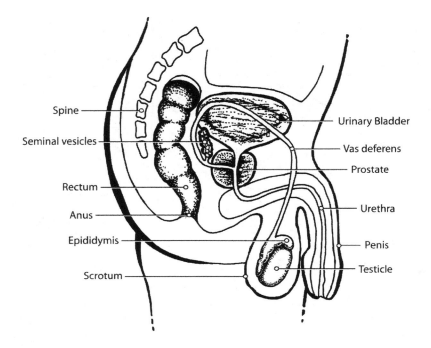

The Prostate and Urination

Prostate illness can interfere with your ability to urinate and in some cases can damage your kidneys and other urinary tract structures. Because the prostate surrounds the urethra, prostate enlargement can squeeze and eventually choke the urethra and make simple urination an agonizing chore.

The urinary tract begins at the *kidneys,* located at the base of the ribs on either side of the spine. These amazing organs are the body's main filters, cleansing impurities from about 45 gallons of water every day. Most of this water is recirculated through the body, producing only two quarts of waste, in the form of urine, in most men.

Prostate Gland Frontal View

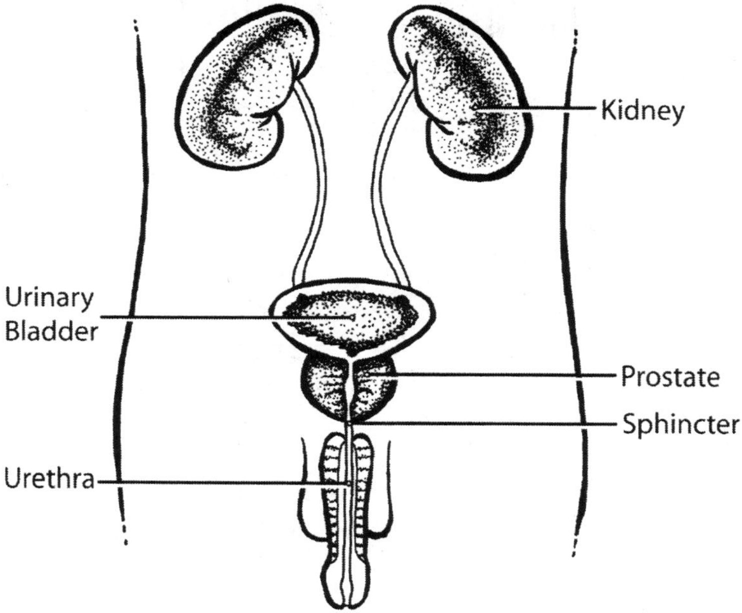

Kidney

Urinary Bladder

Prostate

Sphincter

Urethra

Urine travels to the *urinary bladder* through tubes called *ureters*. The bladder, located above the prostate, holds about a pint of urine. It empties into the urethra, which carries it through a muscle called the *urinary sphincter* and out through the penis. The urinary sphincter is responsible for continence, your ability to contain the flow of urine.

For this marvelous internal cleansing system to help you stay healthy, every mechanism must be in working order. Prostate disorders can harm this delicate balance and keep the structures of the urinary tract from doing their jobs.

Prostate Cancer

Cancer is a collection of cells that are growing out of control. How does this happen? Healthy cells have predictable growth limits and life spans. Not only do cancer cells grow past normal limits, they don't die when they're supposed to. Instead, they divide and spread, sometimes uncontrollably.

A mass of cancer cells is called a *tumor*, but not all tumors are cancerous. A *benign* tumor might grow and squeeze nearby organs, but it does not spread in an aggressive or life-threatening way. Cancer cells, however, can break away from a primary *malignant* tumor site and spread, or *metastasize*, to nearby organs or to distant sites through blood or lymph vessels. Cancer destroys normal tissue and creates new tumors as it spreads.

How does cancer spread through the lymph system? *Lymph* is a fluid that bathes every living cell in the body. You might see this clear fluid escaping when you skin your knee, for example. Lymph fights cancer by draining waste from cells, carrying it through vessels and into lymph nodes, which filter the fluid and remove harmful substances. Sometimes, however, there are more cancer cells than the lymph nodes can handle, and the lymph vessels themselves become vehicles for spreading cancer.

Among men in the United States, prostate cancer is second to skin cancer as the most common cancer and second to lung cancer as a cause of cancer death. One out of six men will be diagnosed with prostate cancer during their lifetime and one in 36 will die from it. Each year in the United States, an estimated 225,000 new cases are diagnosed. More than two million Americans are living with diagnosed prostate cancer right now.

The great majority of these men will survive. Most men with prostate cancer do not die from prostate cancer.

6

Compared to most other types of cancer, prostate cancer grows slowly and offers high potential for cure. Many men with *microscopic prostate cancer* never know they have it and eventually die from unrelated causes.

This doesn't mean you should ignore symptoms or delay seeking treatment, however. Untreated, prostate cancer can spread within the prostate capsule and outward to seminal vesicles, lymph nodes, bones, lungs, liver, and elsewhere in the body.

Typically, prostate cancer starts in the peripheral zone of the gland. Male hormones, especially testosterone, stimulate growth of both normal and cancerous cells in the prostate. Accordingly, testosterone fuels prostate cancer growth.

Symptoms of Prostate Cancer

Early prostate cancer has no symptoms. You could be feeling hale and hearty when you are diagnosed. For many men, the diagnosis comes as a complete surprise.

Malignant tumors in the prostate generally start out very small. It usually takes years for prostate cancers to grow large enough to obstruct the flow of urine. Fortunately, modern diagnostic methods can detect prostate cancer long before symptoms have a chance to develop.

If prostate cancer grows enough to exhibit symptoms, they are much like those of noncancerous prostate disorders. One or more of the following symptoms can indicate prostate cancer:

- Getting up at night to urinate
- Frequent urination during the day
- Weak or interrupted urinary flow
- Difficulty starting the urine stream
- Dribbling

- Urgency
- Leakage
- Pain or burning during urination
- Needing to strain to urinate
- Less rigid erections than normal
- Pain during ejaculation
- Less ejaculate (semen) than normal
- Impotence

Though such symptoms may not indicate prostate cancer, they should never be ignored. Almost any disease, no matter how minor it is in the beginning, can be dangerous if left untreated.

Prostate cancer that has spread beyond the gland itself can cause a range of symptoms, depending on where the cancer is located. Such symptoms include pain, sometimes intermittent, in the back, ribs, hip, or shoulder; fatigue; weakness; and generalized aches and pains. Even though these symptoms are vague and could easily be harmless, don't ignore them. Too many men regard their symptoms, whether difficulty urinating or intermittent aches and pains, as "normal signs of aging." It bears repeating: See your doctor right away if you're experiencing symptoms you can't easily explain.

Risk Factors for Prostate Cancer

All men are at risk for prostate cancer. Heredity and environment can greatly affect the degree of risk.

The risk factors and associated trends and statistics cited below apply to men in the United States. Globally, there are huge variances in prostate cancer causes and prevalence. Men in Australia, the Caribbean, North America, and northwestern Europe have disproportionately high rates of prostate cancer.

Age. Rarely are men under age 40 diagnosed with prostate cancer, but the risk increases rapidly after age 50. Two-thirds of prostate cancers are found in men over 65.

Family history. Up to 10 percent of prostate cancer diagnoses correspond to a family history of prostate cancer or breast cancer. Having a father or brother diagnosed with prostate cancer, especially before age 60, increases risk by 3 to 5 percent over those with no family history. The risk grows if two, three, or more relatives are diagnosed with prostate cancer. A family history of breast cancer is also a factor, particularly in combination with a family history of prostate cancer. Genetic research is continually at work to refine our understanding of heredity's role in prostate cancer risk.

Race and ethnicity. In the United States, African-American men are at the greatest risk of getting prostate cancer and dying from it. Research suggests that diet and other lifestyle factors play a role in this racial disparity. From 1999 to 2010, however, prostate cancer incidence rates as well as death rates declined dramatically for African Americans compared to other groups.

After African Americans, white men have the highest rates of prostate cancer incidence and death, followed by Hispanic, American Indian/Alaska Native, and Asian/Pacific Islander men.

Occupation. Though the evidence is inconclusive, it appears that employment in some occupations places men at higher risk for prostate cancer than the general population—in particular, agricultural workers, soap and perfume manufacturers, leather workers, white-collar workers, mechanics, and welders. With the exception of white-collar workers, these occupations involve exposure to pesticides, herbicides, fertilizers, and other chemicals. Depending on the type, degree, and duration of exposure, toxins may damage cells to the point where they mutate and become cancerous. Exposure to the element cadmium, which interferes with zinc absorption, is also a potential risk. Men with prostate cancer tend to have lower levels of zinc in their bodies.

For white-collar workers at sedentary desk jobs, the risk is linked to inactivity combined with unhealthy lifestyle choices.

Lifestyle. Whether or not you have been diagnosed with prostate cancer, lifestyle factors such as quiting smoking and exercising can improve the quality of your overall health and prolong your life.

If you exercise regularly, keep it up; if you don't, ask your doctor to recommend an exercise plan. Besides its many other benefits, exercise is known to boost the immune system and improve mood and mental balance.

In 2011, results from an ongoing eighteen-year study showed that exercise significantly reduced death rates in participants diagnosed with prostate cancer. Men reported the average intensity and time per week they exercised. Those involved in vigorous activity (more than three hours per week of running, swimming, cycling, etc.) were 61 percent less likely to die of prostate cancer than men who did less than one hour per week of vigorous activity. Light to moderate exercise showed short-term benefits but did not reduce the risk of premature death from any cause.

Men who smoke are more likely to get prostate cancer, to experience a recurrence, and to die of the disease. Former smokers may be similarly at risk, depending on the amount inhaled and the length of time they smoked. Studies do not agree on the specific increase in risk, varying from 10 to 50 percent. Unrelieved stress and smoking are related; either or both create damage at the cellular level. No one doubts smoking's health dangers overall, however. Health experts agree that stopping a tobacco habit is one of the best things you can do for your immediate and long-term well-being.

Preventing Prostate Cancer

For more than a decade, scientists have known that a high-fat, low-fiber diet greatly increases the likelihood of cancer. Over and over, research has shown that a more healthful diet not only decreases the likelihood of cancer, it may slow cancer's growth. A southern Mediterranean diet emphasizing olive oil and cooked vegetables or a rural Japanese diet—high in rice, fish, soy, vegetables, and green tea—may actually prevent prostate and other cancers and reduce the changes of recurrence.

Many doctors recommend that, whether or not you have prostate cancer, fat should account for no more than 20 percent of your calorie intake. To reduce the risk of prostate cancer and other disorders, your daily diet should include at least five servings of fruits and vegetables per day from a variety of sources, minimal red meat, and no more than three servings of dairy products,If you're not sure what constitutes a serving, your doctor can clarify the term.

Most people—apart from those with allergies, food sensitivities, or other conditions with their own sets of dietary rules—will benefit from a variety of wholesome foods, including:

- *Soy products,* such as tofu and soy milk, which may block angiogenesis, the process by which cancer cells create blood vessels on which to travel through the body.
- *Green tea,* which contains *antioxidants* that neutralize cancer-causing *oxidants,* or *free radicals,* in the body.

- *Red grapes, grape juice,* and *red wine,* which also contain antioxidants, though of a different type than those in green tea.

- *Fresh fruits and vegetables,* which may contain beta-carotene (which protects against rapid cell growth), lycopene (an anticancer pigment present in red-colored foods), and antioxidants. In general, the darker the color, the greater the benefit. That gives you a lot of delicious, nourishing foods to choose from, including dark-green leafy vegetables (spinach, romaine lettuce, and other salad greens), cruciferous vegetables (broccoli and cauliflower), beets, carrots, yams, strawberries, raspberries, blueberries, peas, watermelon, and citrus fruits.

- *Fresh herbs,* including oregano, peppermint, rosemary, and thyme, which contain antioxidants.

Meat, eggs, and seafood must be thoroughly cooked. Otherwise, fresh foods are the best sources of nutrition.

Supplements may provide essential nutrients lacking in some diets. Consult your doctor before taking supplements, and ask for recommended dosages in light of prescription and nonprescription drugs you are taking.

Don't take vitamin E supplements if you have a bleeding problem or you're taking blood thinners, and stop taking it several weeks before surgery or a biopsy.

Noncancerous Prostate Disorders

Finally, while we're discussing prostate disorders, let's examine two common noncancerous prostate conditions that can interfere with urination: *benign prostatic hyperplasia (BPH)* and *prostatitis.* These conditions usually do not affect younger men but often develop after a man has reached his 40s. It is important to note that these two conditions do not cause prostate cancer, nor do they place you at greater risk for it.

Benign Prostatic Hyperplasia

Benign prostatic hyperplasia (BPH) is an enlarged prostate. The enlargement comes from small noncancerous (benign) growths (hyperplasia) inside the prostate. In a man with BPH, the prostate might grow from the normal walnut size to apricot size after age 40 and lemon size by age 60.

As the prostate grows, it squeezes the urethra and makes it difficult to pass urine. BPH symptoms include urinary irregularities—frequent or urgent urination, a weak urinary stream, or difficulty urinating, for example. Even so, only about half of men with BPH require treatment. Sometimes, however, symptoms become more than a nuisance. If the bladder is unable to empty properly, urine can back up into the kidneys and impair their essential function, straining impurities from body fluids.

There are drugs on the market for treatment of BPH, but many doctors believe that medication is just a stopgap measure that postpones the inevitable. When BPH is severe, surgery may be needed, usually *transurethral resection of the prostate (TURP)*, which requires no skin incision. Surgeons remove the overgrown prostate tissue with an instrument attached to a slender tube that is inserted through the urethra.

Prostatitis

Prostatitis is inflammation of the prostate. Its symptoms include frequent, difficult, or painful urination; pain in joints, muscles, the lower back, and the pelvis; pain during ejaculation; aches, fever, chills; and blood in the urine.

Acute bacterial prostatitis, caused by bacteria, afflicts many men between 40 and 60 years of age. *Chronic bacterial prostatitis,* different from the acute form by being recurrent and longer lasting, is more often found in men between 50 and 80. Bacterial forms of prostatitis are sometimes referred to as prostate infections.

Nonbacterial prostatitis, which is of unknown cause, occurs most often in men from 30 to 50. Though antibiotics are usually effective against bacterial prostatitis, the nonbacterial form has no known cure. Like arthritis and other chronic ailments, however, nonbacterial prostatitis is treatable with anti-inflammatory drugs.

2 Getting a Diagnosis

If you've been putting off your annual physical or postponing that free prostate screening, don't delay any longer. If found early, prostate cancer is curable, but it tends to become more aggressive as it grows.

A variety of diagnostic tests can help your doctor determine whether you have prostate cancer. Before prostate cancer screening and early detection were available, up to a third of first-time diagnoses found advanced prostate cancer. Today, advanced disease is involved in only about 5 percent of initial diagnoses. Simply put, screening and early detection are lifesavers.

Diagnostic Tests

To screen for prostate cancer, doctors first rely on a digital rectal examination (DRE) and a blood test that measures prostate-specific antigen (PSA). Although preventive PSA screening has been used for years, it is still subject to controversy. Some doctors feel PSA tests should be part of regular check-ups. Others don't, because the tests sometimes falsely come back as positive resulting in unneeded tests and treatments. Most prostate cancers are noninvasive and slow-growing, and most men with prostate cancer die of other causes long before prostate cancer becomes a problem. Many doctors and patients choose not to go through the pain and expense of aggressively treating this cancer unless it causes problems or starts growing quickly.

The American Cancer Society Recommendations:

The American Cancer Society recommends that men make an informed decision with their doctor about whether to be tested for prostate cancer. Research has not yet proven that the potential benefits of testing outweigh the harms of testing and treatment. The American Cancer Society believes that men should not be tested without learning about what we know and don't know about the risks and possible benefits of testing and treatment.

Starting at age 50, men should talk to a doctor about the pros and cons of testing so they can decide if testing is the right choice for them. If they are African American or have a father or brother who had prostate cancer before age 65, men should have this talk with a doctor starting at age 45. If men decide to be tested, they should have the PSA blood test with or without a rectal exam. How often they are tested will depend on their PSA level.

Should I Be Screened?

The timing and tests given at your initial screening can be discussed between you and your doctor. Cancer organizations make differing recommendations for frequency and methods used to test for prostate cancer depending on their approach to analyzing the risks. No matter what your age and risk factors, don't delay seeing your doctor if you're concerned about symptoms.

Some medical experts recommend earlier testing–a PSA blood test with or without DRE–starting at age 40 for African-American men and any man with a family history of prostate or breast cancer, age 45 for other men, and annual screenings thereafter.

Digital Rectal Exam

Though the *digital rectal exam (DRE)* is only a starting place, it often finds growths and other irregularities that might indicate cancer many years before you would notice

Digital Rectal Exam (DRE)

The normal prostate gland is soft and smooth. Most prostate cancers start in the outer "zone" of the prostate gland, and doctors are often able to feel lumps or other changes in the gland when performing a digital rectal exam (DRE).

symptoms. The exam may be slightly uncomfortable, but is very brief and seldom painful.

To perform a DRE, your doctor will insert a gloved, lubricated finger into the rectum. He or she will feel through the back rectal wall for lumps, enlargement, or hard, coarse, jagged, or uneven areas of the prostate that might indicate cancer or another prostatic disease.

The healthy prostate is soft, smooth, and symmetrical, and there is a groove down the middle. If the doctor cannot feel the prostate's groove, the gland is probably enlarged.

This and other abnormalities could indicate prostate cancer or a number of other causes: previous prostate surgery or biopsy; past or present infections; prostatitis, inflammation of the prostate; stones in the prostate; or

BPH, benign prostatic hyperplasia, a noncancerous enlargement.

The location of abnormalities is important. Growths due to BPH tend to be in the central gland, whereas almost three-fourths of prostate cancers start in the peripheral or outer zone, the area closest to the rectum. At least a fourth of prostate cancers, however, begin where the doctor can't reach. That's why the PSA blood test is so important; it often reveals prostate cancer that's not apparent in the DRE. Some experts suggest that you go to the same doctor each year for your DRE, since, in theory at least, that doctor will be more likely to notice palpable changes in your prostate from year to year. If your primary care doctor isn't extremely well informed about prostate cancer or doesn't do rectal examinations, you might prefer to see a *urologist,* a doctor who has special knowledge of the male and female urinary tract and the male reproductive organs.

Prostate-Specific Antigen Test

Perhaps the screening test you've heard about most often is one which measures *prostate-specific antigen,* or *PSA;* these antigens are *biomarkers,* also called *tumor markers,* and are normal substances in blood, other fluids, or tissues. Biomarker fluctuations sometimes indicate cancer.

Think of biomarkers as the measurement marks on your car's dipstick. There's a normal level of oil in your car's engine, just as there are normal levels of the various biomarkers in your body. If you check your car's oil level regularly, you know that a small decrease is probably normal but a big drop means trouble, perhaps a major leak. Checking the oil helps you find problems before there are symptoms, such as alarming knocks or pings from the engine or a blown gasket.

Likewise, checking patients' biomarkers helps doctors spot trouble before symptoms appear. Prostate cancer has several biomarkers, PSA being the most important. If there is a lot of PSA in your bloodstream, it usually means there's some type of prostate disorder. If the PSA level rises quickly over two or three tests, it can indicate a large or fast-growing tumor.

All prostate cells, both normal and cancerous, produce PSA. Small amounts of PSA in the bloodstream are normal. Cancerous cells, however, multiply more quickly than normal cells, producing more PSA, An elevated PSA is a warning that something may be wrong and that more studies are needed. That "something" could be BPH, an inflammation, or an infection; a recent biopsy, catheterization, bladder surgery, or another procedure; or recent activity that "massages" the prostate, such as riding a bicycle or motorcycle. Sexual intercourse can elevate your PSA by as much as 10 percent. To avoid a temporary rise in your PSA that could distort the test results, ask your doctor well in advance what you should do, and not do, to prepare.

If your DRE is normal but your PSA is mildly elevated, your doctor will ask for a urine sample to see if you have a prostate infection. If you do, the doctor will probably prescribe an antibiotic and do another PSA blood test several weeks after you've finished taking the medicine.

Your doctor will check for prostatitis and other benign causes of elevated PSA. If these are ruled out and your retest still shows elevated PSA, further tests are called for, usually ultrasound and a prostate biopsy.

What Is a Normal PSA Level?

PSA is measured in nanograms per liter of blood. A nanogram is so small, one-billionth of a gram, that a very sensitive test is needed to detect it. A normal PSA level is not the same for everyone. It varies, depending on age and ethnicity.

Age	Normal PSA	African American Normal PSA
40-50	2.5 or lower	2.0 or lower
50-60	3.5 or lower	3.0 or lower
60-70	4.5 or lower	4.0 or lower
70 and up	6.5 or lower	6.0 or lower

Not all the experts agree on these guidelines. Some say anything above 4.0 is suspicious regardless of the patient's age. Others advise men to have more studies if the first-time PSA is 2.5 or above.

As mentioned, conditions other than prostate cancer can cause PSA levels to rise. Scientists have found several ways to interpret PSA test results to form a better idea of whether cancer is causing the PSA increase. One of these is called *PSA velocity (PSAV)*, which compares PSA levels over time to see how quickly they are rising. Your doctor may suspect prostate cancer if your PSA rises by more than three-fourths of a nanogram per year.

Your doctor may also refer to *free PSA* when interpreting your PSA scores. PSA is found in two forms in the blood—unattached ("free") or attached to a protein. Free PSA is less likely to indicate prostate cancer than "attached" PSA.

Transrectal Ultrasound–TRUS

If the DRE or PSA indicates you might have prostate cancer, you'll probably have at least two additional diagnostic procedures, a *transrectal ultrasound (TRUS)* and a needle biopsy. Don't worry if these tests are scheduled several weeks after your checkup. Prostate cancer usually progresses slowly, allowing time to run the tests and do the studies that give very important information about the cancer. The more specific that information, the better you and your doctor can choose precisely the right treatment if cancer is found.

For the TRUS procedure, the doctor will insert a lubricated ultrasound probe into the rectum just behind the prostate. Because ultrasound waves bounce off normal tissue differently than off malignant tissue, the TRUS probe creates a picture of the prostate and abnormalities it might contain. The doctor views the picture on a TV screen. TRUS shows the size of the prostate, an important baseline measurement, but it can't see all types of tumors.

Some prostate tumors are distinct lumps, which often show up on TRUS, but other prostate tumors are spread out, and TRUS seldom shows these. As a result, a normal ultrasound could merely mean that you, like most men with prostate cancer, have lesions that are flat or small and scattered *(diffuse)*. Like the DRE, transrectal ultrasound can be uncomfortable. If a man cannot tolerate a clinic transrectal ultrasound because of hemorrhoids or a history of them, TRUS may be performed under anesthesia.

Needle Biopsy

In a *needle biopsy,* a sample of body tissue is removed with a needle. This procedure can find cancer that TRUS might miss. Many doctors do TRUS and a biopsy at the same time. They use the TRUS images on the TV screen to show them where to direct the biopsy needle. This makes the procedure more accurate than was possible when doctors had no guidance other than what they could feel with their fingers.

With the ultrasound probe in place, the doctor can direct the biopsy needle to suspicious areas. Using a high-speed biopsy "gun"—a long, thin, hollow, spring-loaded needle inserted through the ultrasound probe—the doctor removes several, usually 8 to 12, small cores of suspicious tissue. A *pathologist,* a physician who specializes in diagnosing diseases, examines these tissues under a microscope. The pathologist calculates the presence and amount of cancer, its grade (how much it deviates from normal tissue), and how advanced it appears to be.

Sometimes after these procedures, doctors are still unsure whether cancer is present and you'll need to repeat the TRUS and biopsy. If the pathologist is uncertain about the biopsy samples, ask your doctor about sending them to a pathologist who specializes in prostate biopsies.

PCA3 Assay

If your PSA test results are outside the normal range, your doctor may order a *PCA3 assay,* which involves an analysis of a man's urine. This test is more specific for prostate cancer. It is helpful in men with a highly suspicious PSA but a negative biopsy. If the PCA3 assay is highly suspicious for the presence of prostate cancer, your physician may choose to repeat the biopsy or suggest a saturation biopsy.

Saturation Biopsy

If a needle biopsy does not result in the discovery of cancer, but your physician still strongly suspects it, he or she may recommend a newer template-guided biopsy called a *saturation biopsy.* Twenty or more tissue samples are extracted through the *perineum,* the area between the scrotum and the rectum, from the prostate and seminal vesicles.

3-D Global Mapping Biopsy

This specialized type of saturation biopsy uses a precisely segmented map of the prostate and allows up to 80 biopsies, using needles guided by ultrasound technology and inserted through the perineum. Each tissue sample is labeled according to which part of the gland it was taken from. This makes it possible to construct an exact "map" of the cancer's location.

Research shows that prostate cancer is found in 40 percent of men who have saturation biopsies after having at least three previously negative biopsies.

Preparing for a Biopsy

Your doctor will give you instructions prior to your biopsy. Be sure to tell your doctor what prescription and over-the-counter medications and food supplements you're taking.

In general, for at least a week before your biopsy, avoid alcohol and don't take any medicines or food supplements that can thin your blood and interfere with its ability to clot. These substances can include aspirin, ibuprofen (Motrin or Advil), and other nonsteroidal anti-inflammatory drugs (except Tylenol); food supplements containing vitamin E, fish oil, ginkgo biloba, or garlic; and the blood thinner Coumadin. .

To prevent infection, your doctor will prescribe antibiotics. In addition, you'll have a cleansing enema before the procedure.

Most patients tolerate biopsy procedures well, but if you know you have a low pain threshold, talk with your doctor about ways to relieve any pain or discomfort during the biopsy. Don't feel timid about requesting one of the topical or local pain relievers available for this purpose. If you wish to be given intravenous sedation to make you sleep during the procedure, or if you're having a saturation biopsy, the procedure will probably be scheduled in an outpatient surgery center.

After the Biopsy

TRUS and prostate biopsies are generally outpatient procedures. Afterward you'll probably be sore, so it's a good idea to arrange for someone to drive you home. The next day you can do just about anything you feel up to. You'll continue to take antibiotics, so don't drink alcohol during that time. The biopsy results should be available within two or three days.

If these tests show you have prostate cancer, you'll understandably be eager to start treatment. Many patients see their cancer as an enemy to be wiped out at the earliest possible moment. Taking a bit more time to study your cancer, however, is to your benefit. The more you and your doctor know, the better you can decide on the most effective treatment.

At this point, your doctor will investigate your cancer's stage, how far it has spread, and the *grade*–how aggressive the cancer is.

Biopsy Risks, Complications, and Side Effects

Serious side effects from biopsies are rare. Some patients worry that a biopsy could cause the cancer to spread. This possibility is so remote that it should not prevent your having a biopsy. Severe bleeding or infection occurs less than 1 percent of the time. It's normal to find blood in your urine, semen, or stool for a few weeks after a prostate biopsy.

Very rarely, infection after a prostate biopsy becomes serious, moving into the bloodstream and causing a high fever, shaking, and chills. This reaction, called *sepsis,* is a medical emergency. Another rare but serious biopsy complication is a urinary blockage, indicated by pain and the inability to pass urine. Seek medical help immediately if you experience symptoms of infection or urinary blockage.

Staging Prostate Cancer

When your prostate cancer is diagnosed, your doctor will try to determine the *stage* of the cancer—whether and to what extent it may have spread beyond the prostate. The progress of prostate cancers is fairly predictable. All begin as small lesions confined to the gland itself. Without treatment, they may spread first to other parts of the prostate, then to the seminal vesicles, then to the lymph nodes, and eventually to the bones in the spine, ribs, or pelvis, and beyond. The cancer's *clinical stage* is estimated by putting together pieces of evidence gathered from the DRE, the PSA, ultrasound, biopsy, and other tests. The more accurate *pathologic stage* is established when a pathologist examines the prostate gland after it is surgically removed.

There are two staging systems—the *Whitmore-Jewett* and the *TNM*. In the United States, TNM (short for Tumor, Nodes, and Metastases) is used more than Whitmore-Jewett. For more information on these staging systems, see the appendix.

Grading Prostate Cancer

In the mid-1970s, Dr. Donald Gleason developed a grading system to measure the appearance and arrangement of prostate cancer cells viewed under a microscope. How the cells look can tell a pathologist a lot about how aggressive the cancer is likely to be.

Healthy cells are *well differentiated*. It's easy to see the cell boundaries, where one cell stops and another begins. Malignant cells tend to be *poorly differentiated;* their shapes and boundaries are blurry, and the normal structure of the tissue is absent.

To assign a grade to prostate cancer cells, the pathologist looks at the two largest areas of cancer in the tissue sample and assigns *each* of them a number from 1 to 5. The higher the number, the more poorly differentiated are the cancer cells. The two numbers are then added to make the *Gleason score*. The less differentiated (separate) and the more disorganized the cells appear, the more aggressive the cancer and the higher the Gleason score.

Low Gleason scores of 2, 3, or 4 indicate well-differentiated cells with a relatively normal-appearing structure. Gleason scores of 5, 6, or 7 indicate moderately differentiated prostate cancer cells and generally slow-growing cancer. Higher scores of 8, 9, or 10 indicate a more disorganized cell structure—poorly differentiated, more aggressive, and faster-growing cancer cells.

Sometimes a pathologist examining biopsied prostate tissue will see abnormal cells that appear precancerous. This condition is called *prostatic intraepithelial neoplasia (PIN), high-grade prostatic intraepithelial neoplasia,* or *atypia.* If cellular atypia is found on your biopsy, your urologist may recommend repeating the biopsy, since atypia indicates a likelihood of prostate cancer developing within ten years.

To discover whether your prostate cancer is confined to the prostate, your doctor will take into consideration such factors as your PSA, clinical stage, and Gleason score. With this information at hand, doctors try to predict how your cancer might behave. Investigators at Johns Hopkins University, led by Dr. Allen Partin, took this approach one step further. By looking at thousands of prostates that had been removed and matching those to the patient's stage, Gleason grade, and PSA score, they were able to construct what are now called the Partin Tables to predict whether the cancer is confined to the prostate. You may wish to ask your doctor where your cancer ranks on the Partin Tables.

Other Tests and Studies

Your doctor may have access to a great variety of other procedures that offer even more specific information about your prostate cancer to help you choose the best treatment.

Bone Scan

If your PSA is higher than 10 or your Gleason grade is 8 or greater, your doctor might want to do a *bone scan* to determine whether a cancer has spread to the bones. Some doctors recommend it for all prostate cancer patients. A radioactive substance is inserted that is absorbed by your body in areas of rapid bone growth. Cancer cells in the bone stimulate new bone growth, and a special camera sees these areas as hot spots. However, other conditions can show up as hot spots, including arthritis, healed bone fractures, and Paget's disease, a nonmalignant, metabolic bone disorder in which bone cells grow out of control.

ProstaScint

ProstaScint is a tool similar to a bone scan except that it finds hot spots in soft tissue rather than bones. ProstaScint is sometimes used with other imaging techniques, such as a CT scan of the pelvis, PET scans, and bone scans.

CT Scan

For a *computerized tomography scan* (*CT scan,* also called a *CAT scan*), a machine moves around your body to take a circular series of X-rays. A CT scan provides detailed photos of tissues and organs inside the body with much greater accuracy than standard X-ray. The test is painless and noninvasive.

Magnetic Resonance Imaging

Like the CT scan, *magnetic resonance imaging (MRI)* presents a three-dimensional image, but uses magnetic waves rather than X-rays. Painless and noninvasive, it can identify bone abnormalities as cancerous or benign. Like CT scans, MRIs may be performed as inpatient or outpatient procedures. The MRI produces a loud, clanging sound as strong electromagnetic fields are switched off and on. Most patients wear ear plugs or listen to music through headphones during the procedure. The test typically involves 20 to 45 minutes of confinement in a tunnel-like structure. If you tend to be claustrophobic, your doctor might give you a light sedative. Some facilities have open MRI scanners, which aren't totally enclosed.

An *endorectal coil MRI* may be used to provide an enhanced image. During an endorectal coil exam, a slim, lubricated, tubular device containing coiled wires capable of sending and receiving radio waves will be inserted into your rectum. A small balloon is then inflated around the device to prevent shifting. When the exam is finished, the balloon is deflated and the apparatus is removed. Most men find this exam not much more uncomfortable than a digital rectal exam.

A newer MRI scan, the *spectroscopic MRI,* may be helpful in determining the extent of prostate cancer. This MRI is conducted in exactly the same way as the traditional prostate MRI, but in addition to examining soft tissue, it measures the levels of the chemicals choline and citrate in the prostate. It has been found that prostate cancer cells contain more choline and less citrate than normal tissues. Thus MRI spectroscopy can indicate which areas are suspicious for cancer.

PET Scan

For *positron emission tomography (PET) scans,* patients are injected with a sugar solution. Since tumor cells use glucose as an energy source, the sugar solution gravitates to cancerous tissue. As a result, PET scans can locate tumors and can tell how quickly they digest the sugar. The more rapid the digestion, the more likely it is that the cells are malignant.

PET scans are not used routinely in prostate cancer staging, however, since prostate cancer cells are slow growing and less likely to light up on PET scans.

Percutaneous Needle Biopsy (PNB)

In advance of surgery for prostate cancer, many doctors recommend a smaller procedure to sample lymph nodes and examine them to see if cancer has spread. *Percutaneous needle biopsy* extracts tissue from deep pelvic lymph nodes using a long, thin needle inserted through the skin. Placement is guided by a CT scan. If you have a PNB procedure, you'll be given local anesthesia and probably intravenous sedation as well. Plan to take the day off. You'll probably be able to go back to work the next day.

After Diagnosis: Choosing a Treatment Plan

The diagnosing procedures described in this chapter give your doctor important information about the treatment method likely to be most effective. If you have been diagnosed with prostate cancer, you will discuss treatment options with your doctor. As you may already know, the basic forms of treatment include surgery, radiation therapy, hormone therapy, and chemotherapy. Treatment options are based on one's age, general health, and stage of the cancer at the time of diagnosis.

3 Surgery for Prostate Cancer

If you're considering surgery as one of your treatment options, you're in good company. Among men with early-stage prostate cancer, surgery to remove the prostate, the seminal vesicles, and the pelvic lymph nodes is the most widely chosen treatment. Surgery may also offer the best chance for a cure. What does the word *cure* mean in terms of a prostate cancer diagnosis?

Nowadays, oncologists are careful about using the word; however, a man who has had his prostate gland surgically removed is generally considered cured if, five years later, he has no evidence of recurring cancer and his PSA level has not increased.

Are You a Candidate for Surgery?

You're most likely to benefit from surgery to remove the prostate if your cancer is confined to the prostate, you have fairly low-grade disease (Gleason score of 6 or less), your PSA level is 4 or less, you're in your early seventies or younger, and you're in good overall health with a normal life expectancy of at least ten more years. There are, of course, exceptions to this profile. Your case is not exactly like anyone else's. Under certain circumstances, higher PSA levels and Gleason scores, cancer that may have spread to the seminal vesicles, and other unfavorable signs might not automatically exclude you from having radical surgery.

If you believe you might be a candidate for surgery and your doctor doesn't agree, find out why. If you're not satisfied with the answer, get a second opinion. Do your own research and talk to prostate cancer survivors. No reputable surgeon is going to perform a radical prostatectomy if he or she doesn't think it will be beneficial; however, you have the right to know why and to state your case.

Surgical Procedures
Radical Retropubic Prostatectomy

A *radical prostatectomy* is a major operation that usually takes two to four hours. It also requires two to four days in the hospital and several weeks' recovery at home.

The term *radical,* in medicine, refers to a treatment meant to remove the source of an illness. You and your doctor may decide that the retropubic approach is best for you. *Retro* means behind, and *pubis* refers to the pubic area, the lower part of the abdomen.

In a *radical retropubic prostatectomy,* your prostate, seminal vesicles, and pelvic lymph nodes will be removed through an incision in your lower abdomen from just below the navel down to the pubic bone. The lymph nodes will be rushed to the lab and immediately frozen, and a pathologist will examine them for cancer. If there are malignant cells showing that cancer has escaped the prostate, the surgeon will probably not continue with the operation. Surgery is unlikely to remove all the cancer once it has spread, and other options will be better able to treat your cancer.

Some doctors, however, might choose to proceed with surgery to remove the prostate even if the patholo-

Radical Retropubic Prostatectomy

The incision for a radical retropubic prostatectomy is made in the abdomen, starting under the navel and extending to the pubic area.

gist finds cancer in the pelvic lymph nodes. The rationale here is that by removing as much cancer as possible, known as *debulking,* your body's immune system can do a better job of fighting the cancer that remains. Debulking is controversial, however, and most doctors are unwilling to put patients through the rigors of surgery if it is unlikely to remove all the cancer.

There's another reason for proceeding with the operation even if local metastases are found. Your doctor might be cautiously optimistic that a cure is possible—even when cancer has penetrated the prostate wall and may have spread to the seminal vesicles. Treatment in this case involves a combination of radical prostatectomy, radiation to the prostate bed, and adjuvant hormonal therapy. *Adjuvant therapy* is treatment that follows the primary form of treatment.

Nerve-Sparing Prostatectomy

If cancer has not penetrated the prostate capsule, your surgeon may attempt a nerve-sparing prostatectomy, which preserves the neurovascular bundles on either side of your prostate. A few decades ago, these nerves were almost always cut during a radical prostatectomy, and patients had to live with permanent impotence, the inability to have an erection. These days surgeons can often preserve one or both neurovascular bundles. When the cancer appears to be located on only one side of your prostate, the surgeon might leave the nerves intact on the opposite side, if he or she is certain that no cancer cells will be left behind. It is not possible to remove only part of the prostate. Even if only one lobe appears cancerous, the doctor will remove the entire gland.

Radical Perineal Prostatectomy

Using the perineal approach, called *radical perineal prostatectomy,* doctors remove the prostate through an incision in the perineum rather than the abdomen. The perineal approach is less common than the retropubic for at least three reasons: It doesn't permit removal and dissection of the pelvic lymph nodes, it makes the nerve-sparing technique difficult, and the surgeon can't remove as much tissue.

Even though the perineal incision is used rather infrequently, it has advantages: The retropubic incision (in the abdomen) places the prostate and surrounding organs and tissues in plain view and within comparatively easy access. The perineal incision is several inches shorter than the retropubic incision. Also, the perineal surgery is over in as little as an hour and a half, the recovery time is shorter as well, and less blood is lost than with the retropubic approach. Finally, perineal surgery might be

Radical Perineal Prostatectomy

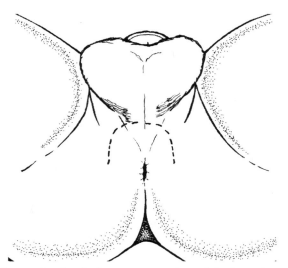

An incision for a perineal radical prostatectomy is made in the perineum, between the scrotum and the anus.

better for obese patients since it provides easier access to the prostate gland.

If you've decided on the perineal approach and your doctor wants to remove the pelvic lymph nodes for dissection, you'll have a separate procedure called a lymphadenectomy. Some surgeons use a traditional surgical approach through a small incision in the lower abdomen. Other surgeons remove the lymph nodes resynthesizing, a less invasive procedure.

Radical Laparoscopic Prostatectomy

Laparoscopic prostatectomy is less invasive than open surgery. It can be used for diagnostic purposes (for example, a biopsy of lymph glands) or, in some cases, for prostate removal. In this procedure, several one-inch incisions are made in the lower abdomen. Using an endoscope, a small viewing tube that contains a video camera with a lens that magnifies the nerves and vessels, the surgeon can see the prostate and surrounding tissues on a screen. A second tubelike instrument able to cut and sew is inserted through another incision. The surgeon removes the cancerous tissue while watching the screen to manipulate the instrument.

The advantages of laparoscopic surgery over open surgery include:

- less pain.
- less blood loss, which is better for the patient.
- improved visibility for the surgeon during the procedure.
- smaller incisions.
- faster recovery—the patient usually goes home the next day, has the catheter removed in about a week, and can resume normal activities within a few weeks.

There are disadvantages as well:

- The surgeon can't actually feel the tissue.
- The tools inserted through the tube have a limited range of motion.
- The screen shows a mirror image of what's happening, which means surgeons need special training using the equipment.

A new type of surgery called *robotic laparoscopic prostatectomy* has become very popular. As with traditional laparoscopic prostatectomy, instruments are inserted through small incisions and the surgeon watches the procedure on a video screen. Instead of the surgeon, however, a robot manipulates the instruments using very tiny robotic "hands." The affected tissue is cut away and the nerves and blood vessels are sewn back together. Unlike the instruments in regular laparoscopic surgery, the hands can turn in all directions and are quite flexible. The computer that interprets the surgeon's movements is able to adjust for tremors or shaking in the instruments, which means the surgery can be much more precise.

Robotic laparoscopy offers the same advantages as regular laparoscopy in terms of minimal pain, minimal blood loss, and faster recovery. In addition, it may be more precise. The surgeon can see the procedure in three dimensions rather than two as with a regular laparoscopy. With robotic surgery the risks are reduced for infection and deep-vein thrombosis. Outcomes are similar to those of open prostatectomy.

Drawbacks include the cost of the equipment (not many hospitals can afford it); the length of time it takes to perform the surgery; and the amount of time and experience a surgeon needs to use it to best advantage.

Current studies indicate that the more procedures a surgeon performs using this equipment, the better the patient's outcome. Today, there are experienced robotic prostatectomy surgeons at most major medical centers. The benefits of robotic surgery include less blood loss, less pain, lower infection rates, less risk of deep vein thrombosis, and shortened recuperative times.

The information below applies to the radical retropubic prostatectomy procedure unless otherwise indicated.

Before the Operation

Your doctor will schedule surgery at least four to six weeks after your needle biopsy or twelve weeks after surgery for benign prostatic hyperplasia. This waiting period will give the prostate and tissues surrounding it a chance to heal from those procedures.

At the time the operation is scheduled, ask whether you should take your regular medications to the hospital when you check in for your surgery and tell your doctor about all prescription and over-the counter drugs, food supplements, herbal products, and other remedies you are taking. The doctor will tell you when to stop taking some or all of these substances before the operation.

For example, seven to ten days before surgery, you'll probably have to stop taking products containing aspirin or ibuprofen, as well as vitamin E, fish oil, garlic tablets, and other potentially blood-thinning substances to prevent excessive bleeding during surgery. If another doctor has prescribed blood-thinning medication for you, let your surgeon know and check with the prescribing doctor before you stop taking it.

Some herbal supplements might interact with the anesthetic given during surgery. Your doctor may tell you to stop taking these products two weeks before your scheduled operation.

Be sure to let your doctor know if you have ever had blood clots. This information helps the anesthesiologist and the surgeon take extra precautions during surgery. To further reduce the risk of blood clots, your doctor will probably have you wear pneumatic stockings during surgery and for a few days after. These stockings improve blood circulation by repeatedly inflating and deflating,.

To guard against infection, you'll start taking antibiotics before the operation and continue for a few days after. Your doctor will advise you to have an enema or take a laxative, or both, the night before surgery and will ask you not to eat for at least twelve hours before the operation begins. You might also be given a special antiseptic soap to shower with before surgery.

Receiving Anesthesia

You'll have a general anesthetic to put you to sleep and possibly an *epidural,* a drip into the epidural space near the base of the spine, to temporarily numb the lower part of your body. The epidural space contains nerves running from your spine to your lower body.

After an injection to numb the part of your back where the epidural will go in—similar to the Novocain shot you get at the dentist—an anesthesiologist will push a long, thin needle into the epidural space. Through the needle, a very narrow plastic tube called an *epidural catheter* will be inserted and the needle itself will be withdrawn. Epidural anesthesia prolongs recovery of bowel functions and sometimes requires an additional day or two in the hospital.

Undergoing Surgery

To perform a radical retropubic prostatectomy, the surgeon will begin by making the incision. The veins that feed the area will be cut and cauterized to achieve what is called a *bloodless field.* Patients rarely require blood transfusions; the few who do usually have large incisions. The average blood loss for an open prostatectomy procedure is 600cc (slightly more than a pint, which represents a single Red Cross blood donation); for laparoscopic procedures, the average amount is 150cc (about 5 ounces or 10 tablespoons).

As mentioned earlier, the surgeon *may* remove the pelvic lymph nodes, which a pathologist will examine immediately. This process, called a *staging pelvic lymphadenectomy,* is sometimes omitted if your Gleason score is lower than 8.

If the pathologist's report shows that your lymph nodes are clear of cancer and the operation continues, the surgeon will remove your prostate, the seminal vesicles, and if needed, one or both neurovascular bundles. In the lab, the pathologist will examine the prostate to determine the cancer's type, grade, extent, and volume. The pathologist will also see whether the *surgical margins* —the edges of the removed tumor—are clear. If not, the finding is called a *positive margin,* meaning that cancer cells were discovered along the edges. A positive margin may predict cancer recurrence, and your physician will discuss additional treatment with you. Pathology results are generally available a day or two after surgery.

The prostatic urethra—the part of the urethra surrounded by the prostate—will also be removed, and the surgeon will reattach the remaining urethra to the bladder neck with sutures. This new connection is called an *anastomosis,* a term worth remembering because you'll need to guard it well in the weeks to come. The surgeon will insert a Foley catheter through the penis to the bladder, anchoring it with a small balloon. While the catheter is in place, urine will bypass the anastomosis so it can heal properly. If the catheter is pulled loose or removed too soon, permanent incontinence—which is otherwise quite rare—could result.

After the Operation

You'll spend an hour or more in the recovery room, where you'll be monitored until the general anesthetic wears off. Very rarely, a patient will have an allergic reaction to the anesthetic used during surgery. Symptoms range from fever or a rash to swelling of the tongue and lips. If you notice any of these symptoms once you become conscious after surgery, be sure to report them without delay. A severe allergic reaction could be fatal.

Cavernous Nerves

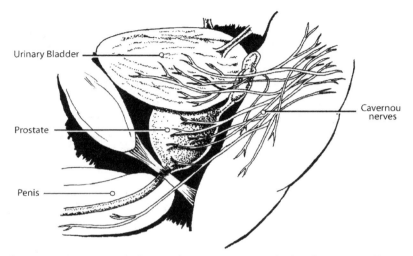

Urinary Bladder

Prostate

Penis

Cavernous nerves

The cavernous nerves, which control erections, are attached to the prostate. These nerves can be easily damaged when the prostate is removed, affecting a man's ability to achieve an erection.

You'll wake up to find several tubes projecting from your body. One or two of them will be drains placed during surgery to suction leakage from the anastomosis. They'll probably be removed before you leave the hospital. As mentioned, the Foley catheter will drain urine from your bladder while the anastomosis heals. You'll have an IV in your arm for fluids and possibly for medication.

Your epidural tube may remain in place for pain relief medication. You'll probably receive a powerful nonnarcotic drug, better than narcotic pain relievers because it's unlikely to upset your stomach. Your pain relief might come in the form of a *PCA pump.* PCA stands for *patient-controlled analgesia,* which means that you control the timing of your pain medication using a device with built-in safeguards against dosing too much or too often. Don't allow anyone else to push your PCA button. If you're too drowsy to do it yourself, you might have too much medication in your bloodstream.

If you have to rely on hospital staff to administer pain medication, don't be timid. You've just had a major insult to the midsection and you have a right to be as comfortable as today's safe and effective medications can make you. The best advice: Don't wait for pain to become intense before seeking pain medication. Try to stay ahead of the pain.

Managing Pain

Gritting your teeth and enduring severe pain can actually interfere with healing and put you at risk for complications. Pain limits your ability to breathe deeply, cough, and move around—all necessary for normal healing. Take pain medications as prescribed rather than toughing it out or waiting until you are having pain.

As mentioned earlier, there is less pain with laparoscopic surgery; the incision is smaller and the incision site is injected with long-acting local anesthetic agents. The less pain you have, the less pain medication you'll need.

Well before surgery, discuss your concerns about pain and medication with your doctor.

Preventing Deep Venous Thrombosis

However capable your surgeon, preventing blood clots in the deep veins of the legs, called *deep venous thrombosis,* requires some effort on your part. It's your job to move about, since mobility keeps your blood circulating so clots don't have a chance to form. Not only are these blood clots painful, they can be deadly. If a clot breaks off and travels through your body, it can move through your heart to a lung. A blood clot in the lung, a *pulmonary embolism,* can be fatal.

You'll be encouraged to walk for a few minutes every hour as soon as you're alert after surgery and for the entire time you're in the hospital. Once you're at home, you'll need to continue this regimen. No need to take a long stroll, which could tire you out. Frequent short walks will go a long way toward preventing blood clots. And don't sit for long on a firm surface with your legs hanging over the edge, which can restrict blood circulation in your legs. Elevate your legs as much as possible.

Recovery at Home

Within two to four weeks you should be able to return to your usual routine, unless that routine is particularly strenuous. Ask your doctor when you can resume heavy lifting, sports, and other vigorous activities. Remember that your body has just undergone a major shock and that your genitourinary system is fragile.

Allowing your body to heal while exerting yourself no more than necessary for blood circulation will be your challenge in the days to come.

Caring for the Foley Catheter

You'll leave the hospital with the Foley catheter still in place and with two bags to collect the urine, a large bag to use at night and a smaller bag taped to your leg for daytime drainage. A tube connects the catheter to whichever drainage bag is in use.

Your doctor might suggest that you limit outings to an hour or so while you're using the Foley catheter. You probably won't feel much like going anywhere for a while anyway, but if you do leave the house, be sure the

Foley Catheter

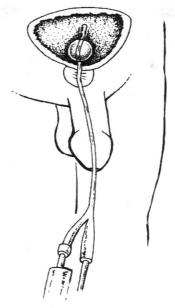

A Foley catheter is used to drain urine from the bladder when normal urination is disrupted. The catheter is threaded through the urinary duct (urethra) and into the bladder.

daytime drainage bag is placed lower than the catheter and is securely taped at all times.

Although the catheter is uncomfortable, it is usually well tolerated. It does require care. Your doctor will give you detailed instructions to follow at home until your two-week checkup, when the catheter will mostly likely be removed. Until then, take showers rather than tub baths and don't get into a swimming pool, Jacuzzi, or sauna.

- Empty the drainage bags often to keep urine from backing up into your bladder—every three to four hours for the leg bag and every eight hours for the larger bag.

- Keep the bags, the tubing, and the connections clean.

- Stay squeaky clean yourself, using soap and water to wash the penis where the catheter exits and the rectal area a few times a day and after a bowel movement.

- Don't pull on the catheter, and be sure there's enough slack in the tube so that you won't pull it out accidentally when turning over in your sleep, for example.

Managing Incontinence

Once your catheter is removed you'll notice some urine leakage. Though it's almost certainly a temporary inconvenience, it can still cause you great embarrassment. Don't drink more than two quarts of water a day for a while and limit caffeine and alcohol to avoid undue stress on the anastomosis, the new connection between the urethra and the bladder neck. Ask your doctor when the anastomosis is likely to be fully healed.

The return of continence is gradual. Meanwhile, your doctor can recommend incontinence products, such as pads or special underwear, you can use to stay comfortable and avoid embarrassment. To help regain control of the urinary sphincter, the muscle that controls the release of urine from your bladder, do Kegel exercises, which involve tightening the sphincter to stop the flow of urine. You can practice these when you urinate, but ask your doctor how to do them properly and how often.

Coping with Impotence

Impotence, or *erectile dysfunction,* does *not* mean that your sex life is over or that it can't be just as exciting and pleasurable as before the operation. If you're in your forties or fifties, you'll most likely regain your ability to have an erection, especially if your surgeon used the nerve-sparing technique, but it will take time. Your doctor can tell you what to expect, and a prostate cancer support group can offer valuable reassurance.

Your doctor might prescribe oral medications such as Viagra, Levitra, or Cialis for erectile dysfunction. Or he or she may recommend a vacuum device a month or six weeks after surgery to improve circulation in the penis.

Two to four months after surgery, if you've been taking erectile-dysfunction medication for a while, your doctor may "prescribe" sexual activity. If you are still impotent, the doctor may begin *penile injection therapy*—actually painless and quite effective.

See chapter 7 for a thorough discussion of strategies for dealing with impotence.

Keeping Bowels Regular

The part of the rectum adjacent to the prostate will be fragile, and you'll need to give it time to heal. It may be a few days after surgery before you have a bowel movement, which should be painless if you take milk of magnesia or use stool softeners, according to your doctor's instructions. Avoid straining, which could injure the rectum.

For three months or so after your operation, do not have an enema or take your temperature rectally. Try to have a bowel movement every day, continuing to take stool softeners and a laxative if necessary, as your doctor recommends. Drinking two quarts of water every day and getting the right amount of dietary fiber can keep you from getting constipated.

Guarding Against Infection

Most of the healing of your incision takes place within six weeks after surgery, but it will continue to heal for up to a year. Infections are very uncommon. If your incision or the IV site on your arm is extremely tender or puffy, tell your doctor right away. Antibiotic medication will usually take care of the problem.

Returning to Normal Activities

Follow your doctor's instructions about what you can do and when. The first week you'll want to take it easy. Catch up on television programs, lay in a supply of good books or crossword puzzles, rest, and drink plenty of fluids. Once you're home, you can probably return to your normal diet as long as it doesn't make you constipated. This would be a good time, however, to change your eating habits if your normal diet is high in animal fat and low in fiber.

The second week you'll feel much better. You might be bored and want to get out and do things. Ask your doctor how much activity is *too* much. Many doctors recommend staying off your feet as much as possible or doing nothing more strenuous than a short walk. You might want to take someone with you on your first stroll to the end of the block, in case you get there and find you're too worn out to get home.

During that second week your bladder may start to rebel against the catheter. You'll experience bladder spasms, annoying cramps that come and go, and probably some urine leakage around the catheter. The best remedy is rest and adequate fluids. Take four to six short walks each day to keep your blood moving without exhausting yourself.

You should be able to return to work after two to four weeks if you have a desk job. Stay home a few weeks longer if your job requires heavy lifting or being on your feet a lot. To give your sutures a chance to heal, don't lift anything over ten pounds for the first six weeks.

Don't drive for at least four weeks, as much for others' safety as for your own. Your reaction time will be slower than before and you might have trouble stopping quickly in an emergency. Your recovery time is shortened if you have had laparoscopic prostatectomy; driving is possible once the catheter is removed.

Wait at least six weeks after surgery to play golf, tennis, bowl, lift weights, or ride a bicycle. Other physical activities can be resumed on the advice of your surgeon.

Postsurgical Doctor Visits

You'll see your doctor a week to ten days after surgery. Your incision will be checked and your sutures and Foley catheter will likely be removed at this time. When the catheter is first removed, you might have *temporary stress urinary incontinence*—urine leakage when you sneeze, for example, or stand up after sitting. Kegel exercises can help.

Two to six weeks after surgery, you'll probably meet with your doctor to go over your pathology report and plan any long-term follow-up care. As often as every three months for the first year and at least once a year thereafter, you will have follow-up visits with your doctor —or doctors, if, for example, you had surgery followed by radiation therapy.

During your postsurgical visits your doctor will likely perform a DRE and a PSA blood test. The doctor will be checking for evidence of recurrence as well as complications from treatment. Your doctor will ask you about any urinary symptoms such as frequent urination, slow stream, leakage of urine, and burning sensations when urinating. You'll also likely be asked about any bowel symptoms such as diarrhea and rectal blood or mucus.

Risks, Complications, and Side Effects of Prostate Surgery

Risks and the possibility of complications from prostate surgery, for the most part low to begin with, are even less likely in the hands of a skilled and experienced surgeon. As you read on, please keep in mind that the percentages are drawn from the entire prostate cancer population.

Some men are more frightened about risks and side effects than they are about the cancer itself. If you are one of these men, please take a minute to consider the statistics.

Risks during or soon after a radical prostatectomy:

- The risk of death is less than one-half of 1 percent.
- The risk of life-threatening complications is lower than 1 percent.
- The risk of incontinence continuing after one year is about 2 percent, although it can continue to decrease for 18 to 24 months after surgery. Around 95 to 98 percent of men will eventually regain some degree of continence. Approximately 70 percent of men will have some degree of stress incontinence that usually resolves over a period of months following surgery. Younger men usually achieve complete continence rapidly due to a well-toned sphincter, while men over age 70 may continue to need one to two pads a day for a longer period of time.

- The risk of impotence is about 30 percent for men in their forties and rises with age to about 80 percent for men in their seventies. Impotence refers only to the ability to have an erection. It does not affect physical sensation or arousal or the ability to have an orgasm. Furthermore, there are several effective remedies for impotence, such as medications and surgical implants. If both nerve bundles are spared, 75 percent of men can expect to return to their previous sexual function. If one bundle is preserved, 50 percent can expect to return to presurgical erectile capability.

- The risk of *urethral stricture* is lower than 10 percent. This narrowing of the urethra is caused by scar tissue that forms after surgery. It can be "stretched" by a urologist in an outpatient procedure.

- The risk of deep venous thrombosis—blood clots in the deep veins of the legs—is about 10 percent, much lower with routine preventive measures such as pneumatic stockings and blood-thinning medication.

- The most common side effect of the epidural is itching. Other epidural side effects, breathing difficulty and infection, are extremely rare.

- Highly unusual after prostatectomy are urinary tract infections, stomach ulcers, pneumonia, and allergic reactions to medication.

- The risk of bowel injury is about one-half of 1 percent. Any such injury can likely be repaired during your operation.

As you can see, the odds are overwhelmingly in your favor, especially if you're younger than 70.

When to Call the Doctor

Call your doctor, call 911, or go to a hospital emergency room immediately if you have nausea, vomiting, difficulty breathing, fever over 100 degrees, chills, a rash, any swelling or redness, or unusual pain, especially in your legs or chest; if you think your catheter is blocked; or if you cough up blood. Some of these symptoms could indicate blood clots, which can be fatal. Treatment with anticoagulant (anticlotting) medication is usually effective when started immediately. If you have these symptoms in the middle of the night, don't wait till morning to report them.

What Is Cryosurgery?

Cryosurgery, also known as cryoablation—"destruction by freezing"—is perhaps best known for its role in skin cancer treatment. Cryoablation has been used since the 1960s to remove skin tumors and precancerous moles. The same principle is at work when cryoablation is used to destroy internal cancers such as those of the prostate. In these procedures, doctors apply supercooled instruments directly to cancerous tissue, killing the cancer but sparing surrounding healthy tissues from damage.

In 2002, the American Urological Association deemed cryoablation of the prostate a "standard" rather than "investigational" procedure. However today, the treatment is rarely used as a primary way to treat prostate cancer. Among other problems, cryosurgery resulted in an impotency rate that exceeded 90 percent.

4 Radiation Therapy

R adiation therapy has come a long way since 1895 when the X-ray was discovered, and since the early part of the twentieth century when Marie Curie published her ground-breaking "Theory of Radioactivity." In your father's or grandfather's day, radiation treatments were less effective than they are now and carried a greater chance of injuring healthy tissue.

Today you have the benefit of higher-energy radiation beams and of beam-shaping devices that target tumors more precisely. Sophisticated imaging studies such as MRI, CT, and PET scans produce multidimensional pictures and allow multidimensional planning and guidance before and during your radiation treatments. Powerful computers record information about your treatments and calculate radiation dosages high enough to be effective but with minimal damage to surrounding healthy cells.

Like surgery, radiation is an aggressive prostate cancer treatment. In fact, radiation therapy is used in more than half of all cancer cases in the United States. If you're a good candidate for radiation, you might be more comfortable with the risks and possible side effects than you are with those of surgery.

Studies indicate that radiation is as effective as surgery for seven to fifteen years. Accordingly, radical prostatectomy is still the preferred curative therapy for younger men, those who could reasonably expect to live for another ten years or more.

It can be tricky, however, to compare the various forms of treatment for at least two reasons. First, treatment technologies are advancing so quickly there hasn't been time for long-term studies to produce solid data on results. Second, the studies that do exist often aren't standardized, measuring different time periods, risk groups, and therapy combinations. Balancing the results can be like comparing apples to oranges. Still, there's solid evidence that men who choose radiation can live for many years after treatment, often without lasting incontinence, impotence, or other troublesome side effects.

Before you decide on a course of radiation therapy for your prostate cancer, talk to others who have had radiation therapy. Discuss your concerns with your doctor, and consider a second opinion from a physician who does not specialize in radiation therapy. You might decide that radiation is indeed the best option for you, but you'll feel better about your decision if you've explored the alternatives.

How Radiation Works

Radiation is effective in killing fast-growing cells. Cancer cells are fast growing. Radiation treatment uses high-energy particles or waves to damage the genetic material in the cancer cells that controls their division and growth.

The goal of radiation therapy is to kill cancer cells while sparing nearby healthy cells. Though some healthy-tissue damage is unavoidable, normal cells are better able to repair the damage than cancer cells.

Radiation therapy is administered by a doctor known as a *radiation oncologist*. There are two types of radiation therapy, *brachytherapy* and *external beam radiation therapy*.

Hormone Treatment before Radiation

It is common for prostate cancer patients being treated with radiation to have hormonal therapy for several months before radiation begins. Any such therapy, given before the primary treatment begins, is called *neoadjuvant therapy*. If your prostate gland is enlarged, your doctor will probably recommend this course of treatment. Neoadjuvant hormonal therapy may also be recommended if your PSA is 10 or higher or your Gleason score is 6 or higher, either of which may place you at moderate to high risk for recurrence.

Hormonal therapy shrinks prostate tissues, both normal and cancerous, by depriving them of testosterone, which they must have to grow and reproduce. The smaller the tumor, the more precisely radiation can be targeted and the less likely the destruction of normal cells. Doctors also believe that hormone therapy helps repair DNA cell damage caused by radiation; this means the hormone treatment increases the kill rate of any cancer cells, making your radiation treatment more effective.

Brachytherapy

One of the two basic types of radiation treatment, *brachytherapy* (BRACK-ee-therapy), also called *seed implantation,* involves the placement of tiny radioactive seeds or pellets directly into the prostate gland. The prefix *brachy-* comes from a Greek word for "short" or "nearby," here referring to the seeds' nearness to the cancerous tissue. You may also come across the term *interstitial brachytherapy*. Interstitial means "within the tissues," in this case, within the prostate gland.

Permanent Seed Implantation

There are two types of brachytherapy, *temporary* and *permanent seed implantation (PSI)*. The latter, in which the implanted seeds are not removed, is the more common procedure. Once implanted, over the ensuing days, weeks, and months, the seeds release radiation that destroys nearby cancer cells. After a period of months, the radioactivity decays.

Temporary Seed Implantation

The less common type of brachytherapy is *temporary seed implantation*, also called *high-dose-rate (HDR) brachytherapy*. The procedure uses highly radioactive pellets that are not left in the body. HDR brachytherapy can deliver more intense radiation than permanent seeds and may be more advantageous to men in higher risk categories. The higher the radiation dose, the more effectively it destroys cancer cells; but a dose that is too high can inflict excessive damage on healthy tissue and create undesirable permanent side effects, including severe bowel and urinary problems.

HDR has several advantages over permanent seeds. The higher-dose radiation can be more powerful against cancer. Also, the distribution of the radiation dose near the urethra can be optimized without increased risk of injury to the urethra. Since most of the data on long-term effectiveness of brachytherapy comes from permanent seed implants, however, most radiation oncologists still prefer PSI.

Before Brachytherapy

Preparing for brachytherapy is similar in many ways to preparing for radical prostatectomy. Usually, you'll wait eight to twelve weeks after you begin hormonal therapy

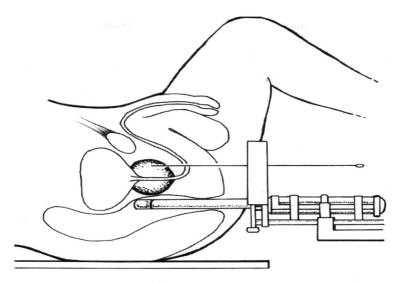

During a seed implant, an ultrasound probe, inserted in the rectum, helps the physician guide needle-like instruments in the prostate, where the radioactive seeds are delivered.

to give the prostate a chance to shrink. You'll also start taking antibiotics ahead of time to prevent infection. As with surgery, you'll be told when to stop taking drugs or supplements that might make your treatment more difficult or risky. Some doctors tell their radiation therapy patients to stop taking antioxidant supplements (vitamins C, E, and selenium), which may interfere with cancer cell destruction.

For both permanent and temporary brachytherapy, seed placement will be planned and dosages calculated in advance with X-rays, CT scans, ultrasound, PET scans, or other imaging techniques. Two to six weeks before seed implantation, you may also have what is called a *planning study* performed on an outpatient basis. During this study, the doctor will insert an ultrasound probe through the rectum; an enema the night before will provide a clear field of view. The probe will project images onto a television monitor. The computer software has a superimposed grid to help the doctor determine where to implant the radioactive seeds.

Your doctor might also schedule an electrocardiogram (EKG), blood tests, and a chest X-ray. These tests help your doctor decide what kind of anesthetic to use. You may also have a *staging pelvic lymphadenectomy,* a brief operation to sample the pelvic lymph nodes and examine them for cancer. If the procedure finds that cancer has spread, your doctor will probably recommend a treatment such as hormonal therapy.

Your doctor may prescribe a blood thinner if you have a history of blood clots and the doctor determines it will not cause excessive bleeding. Just prior to your brachytherapy treatment, your doctor might also prescribe a steroid to prevent swelling from the procedure. You will probably be instructed to have an enema the night before your radiation treatment and to eat nothing after midnight.

Delivery of Permanent Brachytherapy

The procedure to insert permanent radioactive seeds takes about an hour. You'll probably check in to the hospital the day of the procedure, which will be done under general anesthetic or local anesthetic with sedation. Many patients receive an epidural anesthetic to numb them from the waist down and possibly a sedative to make them relaxed. A Foley catheter will be inserted and you may have intravenous antibiotics during the treatment.

In years past, nothing but eyesight and instinct guided doctors in seed placement. Today, doctors use high-

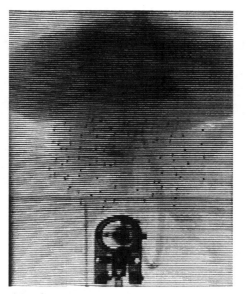

This X-ray was taken after brachytherpay, in which several dozen radioactive seeds were implanted in the prostate gland.

tech imaging equipment and computer software to localize the prostate, determine where to place the seeds, and calculate dosages.

To begin the implantation, the doctor will insert an ultrasound probe into the rectum. The ultrasound probe projects images onto a TV monitor to ensure precise seed placement. A perineal template, attached to the probe, has a grid with tiny holes in it. This grid is sutured to the perineum. Long, thin needles are then used to guide catheters through the template holes and into the prostate gland, where the radioactive seeds are implanted. Between 50 and 100 seeds are inserted. Each seed is about the size of a grain of rice. Rows of seeds are deposited uniformly throughout the prostate so that the radiation can cover the entire gland.

Delivery of Temporary Brachytherapy

The procedure to insert temporary seeds is similar to that of implanting permanent seeds. It differs in that the temporary seeds are not left in the prostate and the entire procedure takes a day or two.

For a temporary seed implant, between 20 and 49 narrow plastic catheters are guided into the prostate. The number of catheters inserted depends on the size of the prostate gland, with a larger gland requiring more catheters to treat a larger volume of tissue. These catheters remain in place 24 to 36 hours to accommodate two or three treatments. During a treatment, one radioactive seed travels in and out of each catheter. A computer program "instructs" the seed where and how long to dwell in any position in the catheters.

After Brachytherapy

After either form of brachytherapy, you'll spend an hour or more in the recovery room until the general anesthetic wears off. The Foley catheter will probably be removed if you have had a permanent seed implant. You'll be given pain medication, and you'll probably receive oral antibiotics to take for several days. Generally, you'll go home that day or the next, and you'll be able to resume most of your activities right away, including going back to work.

After permanent seed implantation, you should wait four to six weeks before having sex, using a condom for as long as your doctor recommends. Some men who have had permanent implants are concerned that they might be "radioactive." It's very unlikely that the radiation could harm others you come into contact with. To be on the safe side, however, avoid close contact with babies, small children, and pregnant women for several weeks after treatment. As an additional precaution, underwear that is lined with lead may be worn for two months following the procedure.

Follow-Up Visits to Your Doctor

After brachytherapy, you'll need to see your radiation oncologist every three to six months for a DRE and a PSA blood test. As in all follow-up visits, doctors are being vigilant, watching for any signs of cancer recurrence or complications from treatment.

If you've had permanent seed implants, your doctor will probably do a CT scan a few days to a month after treatment. Your doctor will check for any cold spots, areas that the seeds are not reaching with radiation. If a cold spot is discovered, additional seed implants are unlikely. Instead, the doctor may wish to monitor the cold spot for a time or supplement the original treatment with external beam radiation, provided that the radiation dose to the rectum does not exceed its tolerance. The five-year survival rate does not seem to be adversely affected by a cold spot.

External Beam Radiation Therapy

The other basic type of radiation therapy is *external beam radiation,* also called *EBRT* or *XRT.* This painless form of treatment uses radiation beams from outside the body to destroy cancers. Treatments typically are given five days a week, Monday through Friday, over a seven- to eight-week period. Weekend breaks are important, giving normal cells a chance to repair themselves.

For well-chosen radiation candidates, EBRT can be as effective and as safe as seed implantation. In part, that's because newer techniques allow much greater precision than conventional EBRT, which uses lead blocks to keep

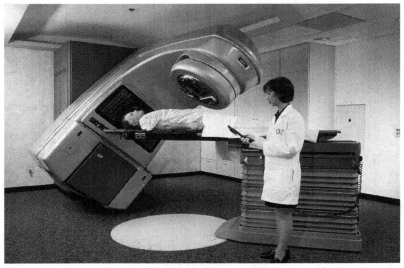

This photo represents a man undergoing external beam radiation therapy.
Photo courtesy of Varian Medical Systems of Palo Alto, California

radiation from damaging the rectum, bladder, urethra, and other structures.

Before External Beam Radiation

Prior to starting treatments, you may have a simulation, or planning session, in which the doctor outlines the radiation target and a physicist develops a radiation treatment plan. The simulation process takes about 20 minutes.

You'll lie on a simulation couch—a narrow, rectangular table—and after you're injected with iodine contrast material, a CT scan will identify your prostate and surrounding tissues. The area to be treated will literally be drawn on your body with a marker, and tiny permanent ink tattoos will be placed in the corners and/or center of the area. It's important that you remain absolutely still during your treatments. To keep your body from moving, an immobilization device will be prepared. The device might be a bag filled with a chemical that turns to Styrofoam and conforms to your shape when you lie on it. Alternatively, you might lie on a bag filled with Styrofoam pellets while technologists form a mold by suctioning out the air with a machine similar to a vacuum cleaner.

To be sure you're completely familiarized with the treatment process, you'll have a dry run before your first treatment.

Delivery of External Beam Radiation

When it's time for your treatment, you'll be asked to empty your bladder, then you'll undress from the waist down and cover yourself with a gown and a towel as you lie down on a table. Radiation therapy technologists may spend ten minutes or more arranging your body in the correct position as directed by the tattoos to make sure the radiation is focused precisely on the target.

The prostate gland can change position, according to the fullness of the bladder and rectum. To address shifts in prostate position, some radiation therapy centers use *BAT,* which stands for *B-mode acquisition and targeting.* This is a special ultrasound-based locating system designed to maximize the precision of external beam radiation. The B-mode system indicates whether the technologist needs to make subtle shifts in the treatment table position, based on tumor location pinpointed by ultrasound.

Unlike brachytherapy, EBRT requires no incision or anesthesia. You'll simply lie still while radiation beams are directed at your prostate and the surrounding area. The treatments themselves last five minutes or less. You won't feel anything on your skin, and all you'll hear is the whir of the EBRT machine, called a *linear accelerator*—a high-energy X-ray unit that moves around your body sending precisely calculated doses of radiation to the tumor.

As you enter the latter weeks of treatment, you might feel tired, but you'll regain your normal energy shortly after the treatment ends. Since external beam therapy is painless, there's no need for pain medications.

Three-dimensional conformal radiation therapy (3D-CRT) uses CT scanners and computers to track the position of your prostate and focus the radiation. The more precisely radiation can target the cancer the less likely it is to damage nearby tissue, nerves, or organs. Cancer is usually an irregular shape, so precision is key. One type of 3D-CRT is *intensity-modulated radiation therapy (IMRT);* this method of treatment sends multiple radiation "beamlets" coming from many directions that combine to accurately target the cancer site Each IMRT treatment takes about twenty minutes.

Other new variations of EBRT may differ from the conventional approach according to what kinds of radiation particles are used. Proton and neutron beam therapies are promising but not yet widely available. They use a different type of radiation but have the same effect. Physicists, radiologists, and surgeons are inventing new procedures as computer-aided technology changes the way prostate cancer is diagnosed and treated. Newer cancer treatments aim to reduce pain, limit side effects, and target cancer cells throughout the body instead of removing them through surgery.

Several newer radiation treatments hold promise in treating low-risk prostate cancer that hasn't spread. *Stereotactic body radiotherapy (SBRT),* also called *Cyberknife,* uses finely focused radiation to destroy tumors and stop growth. A computer-controlled "robot" corrects radiation beams during treatment for any patient movement. Because the highly focused radiation can heat the tumor to high temperatures without affecting surrounding tissue, SBRT can usually be given in about five treatments versus daily treatment over several weeks for other radiation therapies. There is no long-term data on SBRT for the treatment of prostate cancer, though early data look promising.

Image-guided stereotactic radiosurgery (SRS) is similar to SBRT but is believed to be as effective as surgery. Radiation is used to kill the cancer cells, which are then absorbed into the body and eliminated as waste. SRS may prove useful in men who can't have surgery or whose prostate cancer has been diagnosed at an early stage. The first five-year study, although limited, shows recurrence rates similar to those after surgery. SBRT and SRS are not yet widely available.

After External Beam Radiation

Since external beam radiation treatment does not require an incision, the recovery time is shorter than after brachytherapy. Some fatigue is likely, since your body will have experienced major insults. Many doctors believe that the fatigue associated with radiation is as much a result of psychological stress and sleep deprivation (from nighttime urination and hormone-induced hot flashes) than of the radiation itself.

Once your treatment is completed, your doctor will ask you to schedule follow-up visits every three to six months. As with other follow-ups, you will have blood drawn for PSA testing and DRE.

Are You a Candidate for Radiation Therapy?

Radiation treatment is best suited to patients whose cancer is confined to the prostate. It can be a good alternative to radical prostatectomy for older men or for those who are not robust enough to undergo invasive surgery.

Men with large tumors or enlarged prostate glands are not the best candidates for radiation, though pretreatment with hormone therapy may shrink the tissues enough to make radiation an option. EBRT is a better option than brachytherapy if you've had a TURP (transurethral resection of the prostate) procedure for benign prostatic hyperplasia. Why? Because if the prostate gland has been "hollowed out" with a TURP procedure, there is usually not enough tissue to anchor the radioactive seeds. And because external beam therapy can be directed to the prostate, seminal vesicles, and pelvic lymph nodes, it can cover a larger area than seed implantation, which is usually restricted to the prostate itself.

For EBRT, a major consideration is whether there is a treatment center near you, especially one that offers the newer 3D conformal or IMRT. If not, you're looking at the time and expense involved in commuting to a regional center or finding lodging for two months or so. The typical EBRT schedule—Monday-through-Friday treatments for up to eight weeks—is a key part of the treatment's effectiveness. You can't, for example, take a few weeks off in the middle.

Brachytherapy alone is usually recommended for those patients who are at low risk for recurrence. Patients with PSAs over 10, Gleason scores of 7 or above, and extensive cancers on both sides of the gland will usually be offered a combination of brachytherapy and EBRT.

Risks, Complications, and
Side Effects of Radiation Therapy

Most men tolerate radiation therapy well. Lasting side effects are uncommon. The risk of death or life-threatening complications is very low with any form of radiation therapy. Still, it is important to be aware of potential side effects.

The conditions listed below may occur after brachytherapy or, more commonly, external beam radiation therapy. Whatever form of radiation you've been treated with, report all uncomfortable or alarming symptoms to your doctor, who can offer remedies ranging from diet changes and medication to brief outpatient surgery.

Recurrence or Metastases

The greatest complication from radiation therapy is local recurrence or metastases after seven to ten years. Even radiation's strongest advocates say that radical surgery is the best treatment for healthy men in their sixties or younger—men who could reasonably expect to live another fifteen years or longer if their prostate cancer is cured.

Incontinence and Impotence

Severe incontinence occurs in fewer than 2 percent of men treated with radiation. Impotence varies greatly immediately after radiation, from 25 to 50 percent among men age 60 or younger. Impotence and incontinence occasionally worsen in the months and years after treatment because irradiated healthy cells may lose the ability to repair themselves. As is the case after surgery, there are a number of effective treatments.

Common Short-Term Complications

For brachytherapy patients, short-term genital problems are common after radiation. Symptoms can include tenderness where brachytherapy needles were inserted, sore testicles or penis, and pain during ejaculation. For both brachytherapy and ERBT patients, other side effects may include urine leakage (temporary incontinence), frequent need to urinate, difficulty urinating, and stinging or burning during urination or bowel movements. You might see blood in your urine, feces, or semen. These problems will probably go away on their own within a few weeks after treatment, but be sure to mention them to your doctor.

If urinary retention is acute, you'll feel bladder pressure but won't be able to urinate. Up to 15 percent of men require a Foley catheter for four to six weeks after radiation.

Men who have had ERBT may experience diarrhea as a side effect.

Urethral Stricture

With both forms of radiation treatment, there is a slight risk of urethral stricture, a shrinking of the urethra caused by scar tissue. A physician can "stretch" it back to size in an outpatient procedure.

Rectal Injury

Both forms of radiation treatment carry a risk of injury to the rectum. The first sign of such injury is often blood or mucus in the stool. Usually such injury can be repaired with laser surgery or cortisone-containing suppositories or enemas. If damage is severe, which is rare, major surgery may be necessary.

Infection

Occasionally the prostate can become infected shortly after permanent or temporary seed implantation, requiring treatment with antibiotics.

Expelled Seeds

Rarely, seeds work their way out of the body through urine or semen (one of the reasons it's important to use a condom for a few months). If this happens, do not touch the seeds. Pick them up with rubber or vinyl gloves, wrap them securely in several layers of newspaper, and discard the gloves and the seeds in an outdoor trash container with a tight-fitting lid. The amount of radiation emitted is unlikely to be harmful, but you want to be sure that children or animals do not come in contact with the seeds. If you should expel a seed into the toilet, simply flush it. Retrieving it would likely mean greater exposure to radiation. Flushing one seed will not harm the environment.

PSA Bump

More than a third of men treated with brachytherapy experience a PSA bump eight to ten months after radiation. This temporary PSA elevation is almost always due to prostatitis, or prostate inflammation, rather than recurrent prostate cancer.

Other Types of Radiation Treatments
Combination Treatments

Your doctor might recommend EBRT or brachytherapy alone or in combination, though brachytherapy is usually combined with EBRT, hormone therapy, or both. EBRT can boost the radiation dosage delivered by permanently implanted seeds. Your doctor may recommend supplementing brachytherapy with EBRT if there's a high risk of cancer outside the prostate but confined to the seminal vesicles and pelvic lymph nodes.

Radiation therapy is not ideal for large tumors. As mentioned at the beginning of this chapter, many doctors prefer to shrink bulky prostate cancer tumors and the prostate itself with hormone therapy before beginning a course of radiation treatment. Hormone therapy accomplishes this shrinkage by depriving the prostate, cancerous and normal cells alike, of the testosterone they depend on to survive and grow.

Radiation and Salvage Therapy

When a treatment fails, either because of local (pelvic area) recurrence or distant metastases, doctors often recommend *salvage therapy*. Salvage treatments may be given in the hope that a cure is still possible, especially if the recurrence is confined to the prostate as suggested by a Gleason score of 7 or lower. Otherwise, salvage treatments can prolong life by controlling if not eliminating the cancer.

Every form of prostate cancer treatment, no matter how skillfully applied, takes its toll on the body, especially on the rectum, urethra, bladder, nerves, and blood vessels in the pelvic region. For that reason, only certain salvage therapies can be tried after other treatments have failed. It's very unlikely, for example, that your doctor would recommend a radical prostatectomy after radiation treatments failed to eliminate the cancer from your body. For one thing, removing the prostate at that point would probably not remove all the cancer. Moreover, the odds of severe incontinence and impotence are much greater than with surgery or radiation alone.

On the other hand, EBRT is a possible salvage therapy if prostate cancer recurs locally after prostatectomy. EBRT can also be used for recurrence after brachytherapy, although it carries an increased risk of irritation or damage to both the urethra and the rectum.

Seed implantation is seldom used as salvage therapy. It is effective only if cancer is confined to the prostate. As mentioned, if the prostate has been removed (or hollowed out with TURP to treat benign prostatic hyperplasia), there's often no good way to anchor the seeds.

Long-term side effects are almost always increased by salvage therapy. There are effective remedies for these side effects, however, and most men are willing to take the risk if there's a chance for a cure or significant remission of their cancer.

Palliative Radiation

In cases of advanced prostate cancer, radiation can lessen pain and ease other symptoms. Patients with diffuse (widespread) bone pain can have injections of *Metastron (strontium-89 chloride)* or another radioactive isotope that seeks out bone metastases. Local EBRT treatments, sometimes called *spot radiation,* are effective for less diffuse metastases.

When to Call the Doctor

Call the doctor right away if you are unable to urinate. This is probably not a medical emergency, but it does require prompt treatment. Also call your doctor if you have any blood or excessive mucus in your stool, or if you experience severe pain.

Call your doctor, call 911, or go to a hospital emergency room immediately if you have symptoms of severe inflammation or infection—nausea, vomiting, fever of 100 degrees, or chills. Though blood clots are even less likely than after surgery, there's a very small chance of deep venous thrombosis—blood clots that could travel from the legs to the lungs—after seed implantation. Symptoms include pain or swelling in the legs, trouble breathing, or chest pain.

5 Hormone Therapy

Hormone therapy for prostate cancer works by depriving prostate cells, both cancerous and noncancerous, of the fuel they need to survive and grow. That fuel is testosterone, most of which is manufactured in the testicles.

Until just a few years ago, most doctors delayed starting hormone treatments until symptoms of advanced prostate cancer had become acute, as with bone metastases, for example. The thinking was that, since hormone treatments couldn't cure the cancer and created undesirable side effects, these treatments were best reserved for *palliative* use—improving quality of life and sometimes giving patients another year or two of survival.

Newer studies have shown that starting hormone therapy sooner adds more years with good quality of life, and that hormone treatments are highly useful as therapies along with radical prostatectomy and radiation. Hormone therapy remains an important palliative treatment as well.

Scientists are rapidly improving hormone therapy for prostate cancer. Some forms of treatment that had fallen out of favor are getting another look as researchers find ways to counteract their side effects. In this chapter you'll read about a few such therapies, not widely used at present, that nevertheless are still or may soon be part of the prostate cancer treatment arsenal.

How Hormone Therapy Works

Because prostate cells, both normal and cancerous, are fueled by *androgens,* specifically testosterone, scientists have long understood the potential of *androgen deprivation* as a way of controlling prostate cancer. Even when cancer has escaped from the prostate itself, the metastases—whether in the lymph nodes, the bones, or elsewhere in the body—are still essentially prostate cancer cells that can't reproduce without testosterone to feed them.

All hormone therapies work in different ways toward the same goal—to keep testosterone from fueling prostate cancer growth. Hormone therapy drugs can break the testosterone production sequence at any level—keeping testosterone from being made in the first place or blocking its entrance into cancer cells at the end of the cycle.

When androgen-dependent cells lose access to testosterone, they stop growing and dividing. As they die off, androgen deprivation keeps them from being replaced. In this case, hormone therapy not only stabilizes cancer growth but also shrinks prostate tumors and the gland itself. If the tumors have been exerting painful pressure on bones or other body structures, that pain is relieved as soon as the tumors start to shrink.

Why then is androgen deprivation not a cure-all for prostate cancer? Unfortunately, as they grow and reproduce, some prostate cancer cells mutate, becoming *androgen independent.* In effect, they "learn" to survive and thrive without testosterone. Why some men develop a small proportion of androgen-independent cells, whereas other men develop many more, is not well understood.

But for those with fewer androgen-independent cells, hormone therapy can work well for many years, even after other treatments have failed. In general, the lower the percentage of androgen-independent cells, the more likely hormone therapy will assist in long-term survival.

Orchiectomy

Among types of hormone therapy, *orchiectomy* or *surgical castration* is one of the fastest acting and least expensive. In a fairly simple procedure, the surgeon makes a small incision in the scrotum, eases the testicles out of their capsules, clamps and seals off the blood vessels with sutures, removes the testicles, and closes the incision. You might not even need general anesthesia. Light sedation and local anesthesia might be all that's required, and you can probably go home the same day or the next.

With the testicles out of commission, in three to twelve hours a man's testosterone drops to *castration level,* the standard against which all other forms of hormone therapy are measured. The adrenal glands, normally responsible for about 5 percent of the androgens circulating through your bloodstream, continue to produce small amounts of testosterone. The significance of those amounts is still being debated. But almost immediately, symptoms such as bone pain begin to subside.

Advantages and Disadvantages of Orchiectomy

On the plus side, orchiectomy is clearly effective, greatly reducing pain and adding years to the lives of 80 to 90 percent of patients. It is inexpensive, whereas hormone injections to achieve the same results can cost hundreds of dollars a month. On the minus side, your body will change in ways you might expect, since the changes mirror those of menopause in women. In addition to impotence, you could experience hot flashes, breast tenderness or enlargement, loss of muscle tone, reduction in sex drive, and even osteoporosis. Fortunately, doctors have safe and effective ways to counteract most of these side effects. There are even strategies, including implants, for dealing cosmetically with an empty scrotal sac.

Orchiectomy: Risks, Complications, and Side Effects

The operation itself carries little risk. If it's done right—under sterile conditions and with the blood vessels properly sealed off—neither infection nor bleeding should be a problem. Keep the incision area clean using a hydrogen peroxide–water solution followed by an antibiotic ointment such as Bacitracin. Be alert to signs of infection such as unusual tenderness or redness, or pus seeping from the incision. In the extremely unlikely event of excessive bleeding, the scrotum will become enlarged, dark purple, and painful. If this happens, call your doctor, get to a hospital, or call 911, whichever gives you the quickest access to emergency medical treatment.

Recovery from orchiectomy is generally rapid. You'll be advised to avoid heavy lifting, straining, and immersion (no swimming, tub baths, or hot tubs) for one or two weeks.

Chemical Castration

Understandably, many men consider orchiectomy somewhat drastic and opt for *chemical castration,* also called *medical castration,* which can reduce testosterone to castration level within hours or days after treatment starts. Like orchiectomy, chemical castration disconnects the testosterone pipeline, but it uses drugs rather than surgery to do so.

LHRH Agonists

Drugs known as *agonists* stimulate the action of a cell, drug, or hormone. Used in the treatment of prostate cancer, a *luteinizing hormone-releasing hormone (LHRH) agonist* works at the brain level, basically fooling the pituitary gland into stopping production of the hormones that stimulate the testicles to make testosterone —*luteinizing hormone (LH)* and *follicle-stimulating hormone (FSH)*. Usually delivered by injection every three to twelve months, LHRH agonists are currently the preferred therapy for metastatic prostate cancer. Castration level is usually achieved within three to four weeks.

> **Hormone Therapy Agents**
>
> - *Bicalutamide* (Casodex)
> - *Flutamide* (Eulexin)
> - *Nilandron* (Nilutamide)
> - *Zytiga* (Abiraterone)
> - *Enzalutamide* (Xtandi)
> - *Leuprolide* (Lupron)
> - *Goserelin* (Goserelin Acetate)
> - *Firmagon* (Degarelix)

For the first few days after injection, there's actually a surge, called a *flare,* in testosterone production. Flares temporarily enlarge the prostate and any androgen-dependent tumors and can aggravate prostate cancer symptoms. Flares are short lived, however, and are usually harmless for men whose symptoms are not advanced. In men whose symptoms have become distressing and potentially dangerous—bone pain, spinal cord compression, or bladder obstruction, for example—LHRH agonists may be too risky. Orchiectomy or other forms of hormone therapy are likely to be more beneficial for these men.

In general, however, studies have shown LHRH agonists to be as effective as orchiectomy in patients with metastatic prostate cancer who are not susceptible to flare. Other types of hormone therapy can be combined with LHRH agonists to minimize flare.

LHRH Antagonists

Just as an agonist stimulates a cellular action, an *antagonist* blocks an action. Newer drugs, *LHRH antagonists,* block male hormone production and are intended to prevent prostate cancer growth. They appear to lower testosterone levels more quickly than LHRH agonists and do not cause tumor flare. Studies are in progress to find out whether these drugs work as well as LHRH agonists in managing prostate cancer.

Antiandrogens

This class of drugs works by saturating androgen receptors in the prostate, blocking the access of *dihydrotestosterone (DHT)* and testosterone to those receptors. Nonsteroidal antiandrogens don't do as good a job of achieving castration level as other drugs, but given for a week or so before LHRH agonists they can reduce or eliminate flare. Accordingly, antiandrogens are most often given in combination with LHRH agonists rather than alone.

A side effect in men is breast enlargement and tenderness, known as gynecomastia. It is preventable with low-dose radiation to the chest before hormone treatments begin. If you're being treated with an antiandrogen and you develop diarrhea, your doctor will likely reduce the dose.

Estrogens

Estrogen, a sex hormone that regulates women's reproduction, has fallen out of favor as a prostate cancer treatment. Its advantages, however, keep researchers in the chase, looking for ways to harness the drug's benefits without all the drawbacks.

In men, estrogen mimics testosterone in the feedback loop. In other words, when estrogen masquerades as testosterone in the bloodstream, it "fools" your brain. The pituitary "thinks" that your testosterone levels are adequate and cuts back production of the testosterone-stimulating hormones LH and FSH. Testosterone then drops to castration level.

Hormone therapy with the synthetic estrogen *diethylstilbestrol (DES)*, as well as other forms of estrogen, once showed great promise in prostate cancer treatment. DES is inexpensive and conveniently available in tablet form. Unfortunately, at doses high enough to be effective against cancer, estrogens carry unacceptable cardiovascular risks, including heart disease, strokes, and blood clots. Though estrogen therapy for prostate cancer is seldom used (except to alleviate hot flashes, as discussed below), scientists are seeking ways to combine estrogen with other substances that could neutralize the risks.

Estrogen treatment is sometimes grouped with other endocrine therapies, all of which have at least some effectiveness against both androgen-independent and androgen-dependent prostate cancers. Among them are *P450 enzyme inhibitors (Ketoconazole, HDK)*, which disrupt hormone production. These therapies are controversial because of potentially dangerous side effects such as liver damage.

Drug Combinations

Encouraging results have been seen with hormone-therapy combinations such as the *combined androgen blockade*—nonsteroidal antiandrogens used with orchiectomy or LHRH agonists. This makes sense, since only such combinations stop testosterone production in adrenal glands *and* testicles. To date the results of this *combined hormonal therapy* have been impressive.

Intermittent hormone therapy is just what it sounds like—on-again, off-again treatments that are stopped and started based on decreases and increases in PSA levels or troublesome symptoms. Some patients have done well enough after a year of hormone therapy to stop treatments for up to four years before resuming. During this treatment break, men generally become free of the side effects— bone loss, impotence, gynecomastia, hot flashes, and others—that can accompany hormone therapy.

Are You a Candidate for Hormone Therapy?
According to recent evidence, you might well benefit from hormone therapy under any of the following conditions:
- You want to buy time to consider your treatment options.
- You want to decrease the tumor volume before radiation therapy or cryoablation.
- You absolutely refuse to consider invasive treatments such as surgery or brachytherapy.
- Your PSA rises significantly after surgery or radiation.

Hormone therapy can also be a primary treatment in older men who may not be strong enough for invasive treatment or who have widespread metastatic disease.

Hormone Therapy: Risks, Complications, and Side Effects
Since not all hormone treatments work the same way, side effects may differ. You might experience impotence, lower sex drive, fatigue, increased cholesterol, hot flashes, anemia, gynecomastia, osteoporosis, emotional changes, and difficulty concentrating. Your voice will not

get higher, contrary to myth, nor will hormone therapy regrow the hair on your head. Most of these side effects disappear or lessen after you stop hormone therapy.

Osteoporosis can take inches off your height and make your bones so brittle they break easily. A new class of drugs called *bisphosphonates* (including Fosamax, Actonel, Aredia, and Zometa) are particularly effective in fighting osteoporosis and may prevent bone metastases.

Gynecomastia, as mentioned earlier, can be prevented with low-dose radiation, although this treatment has little effectiveness *after* starting hormone treatment.

Hot flashes can be relieved by low doses of estrogen, pills or patches, without causing cardiovascular problems.

Most of these side effects are more uncomfortable or inconvenient than they are dangerous, and most can be alleviated with medication or alternative types of treatment. On the other hand, if you have cardiovascular problems to begin with, if you have liver damage, or if you have metastases that could be dangerously aggravated by the flare phenomenon of LHRH agonists, you will want to approach hormone therapy with caution and frequent monitoring.

Ask your doctor whether hormone treatment would help you as an adjuvant or a neoadjuvant therapy. For example, in advance of radiation as primary therapy, pretreatment with hormones for up to eight months might make radiation more effective by shrinking the prostate and the cancer itself.

Hormone Treatment for Metastatic Castration-Resistant Prostate Cancer (mCRPC)

Most prostate cancer can be kept in check for many years after an initial diagnosis. But sometimes the cancer returns, spreading to nearby tissues, lymph nodes, bones, and other parts of the body. Cancer that grows outside the prostate gland is referred to as *advanced* or *metastatic prostate cancer.*

Metastatic Castration-Resistant Prostate Cancer (mCRPC) is the most challenging type of advanced cancer. It occurs when malignant cells continue growing despite previous surgery, radiation, or drug therapy to suppress male hormones that would fuel them. Instead, residual amounts of testosterone, in particular, begin feeding the cells so they spread. This process can develop many years after a man has been treated initially for nonmetastatic prostate cancer.

Metastatic CRPC is also referred to as *hormone insensitive* because it no longer responds to testosterone-halting treatment. That makes it different from another form of advanced prostate cancer, called *hormone sensitive,* which does respond to continued standard hormone- or androgen-deprivation therapy. Even though cancerous cells have spread, the therapy still improves urinary function and pain control.

With mRCPC, however, physicians must use other approaches to slow any spread of the disease while treating its symptoms. New chemotherapies, immunotherapy, and emerging drugs—*hormone antagonists* or *secondary hormone manipulations*—can delay progression and extend quality of life, if only by months. Your urologist and oncologist may employ several options, based on the progression of the cancer and how it responds. Although there is no cure for any form of advanced prostate cancer, particularly mCRPC, scientists continue to look for ways to halt the disease, improve symptoms, and extend quality of life.

How Does Your Doctor Choose Treatment for Metastatic CRPC?

Treatment for metastatic castration-resistant prostate cancer, the most stubborn type of advanced disease, focuses on delaying the spread of cancerous cells as much as possible while alleviating symptoms.

Your therapy begins even before you have symptoms or radiological evidence of the disease. A rising PSA may be the first indicator of potential mRCPC. At that point, you'll likely undergo standard *hormone* or *androgen deprivation therapy (gonadotropin-releasing hormone [GnRH] agonists and antagonists* plus androgen receptor blockers) to arrest testosterone development.

Once a CT scan reveals evidence of metastases, however, you'll need other help in controlling the cancerous cells. In addition to hormone therapy, your physician may prescribe a new agent from a treatment family known as *immunotherapy.* It's designed to jumpstart your immune system so it can fight the cancer. With this approach, immune cells taken from a sample of your blood are treated in a lab to seek and destroy cancerous cells. The resulting tailored vaccine, known as Sipuleucel-T *(Provenge),* is administered intravenously three times at one- or two-week intervals.

Provenge has proven effective in keeping symptoms to a minimum at least for several months. But if the cancer progresses, causing increased pain in your bones as well as other problems, your doctor will recommend a different treatment course that could include chemotherapy with docetaxal *(Taxotere)* or other chemotherapy agents discussed in chapter 6; secondary hormone manipulations with enzalutamide *(Xtandi)* and abiratorone acetate *(Zytiga);* or both chemotherapy and secondary hormone manipulations. Each approach is designed to improve and extend quality of life for late-stage cancer.

Secondary Hormone Manipulations (Hormone Antagonists)

Secondary hormone manipulations are new drugs used specifically for advanced or metastatic castration-resistant prostate cancer. They stop the growth and spread of cancer by manipulating testosterone in different ways so it can't feed cancerous cells.

The Food and Drug Administration has approved enzalutamide *(Xtandi)* and abiratorone acetate *(Zytiga)* for use specifically after chemotherapy with an agent called docetaxal *(Taxotere)*. (Zytiga is also approved for pre-chemotherapy use; Xtandi may be shortly.) If docetaxal becomes ineffective, your oncologist can choose additional chemotherapies or secondary hormone manipulations.

Zytiga and Xtandi utilize slightly different mechanisms to achieve similar results. Zytiga is known as an *androgen synthesis inhibitor,* meaning it stops the growth of cancerous cells by blocking an important enzyme, CYP-17, that helps in the production of testosterone. Referred to as an androgen receptor inhibitor, Xtandi works by interfering with testosterone binding to prostate cancer cells receptors necessary for cancer cell growth.

Since both are once-a-day oral medications (Zytiga as a tablet and Xtandi via four capsules), you can take them at home or under the supervision of your urologist rather than an oncologist. Although both drugs can cause mild to severe side effects, only Zytiga must be given with twice-daily doses of Prednisone.

In either case, they've have been shown in clinical studies to delay the progression of the disease and the need for chemotherapy.

Your Bone Health

During treatment your doctor will be very concerned about the health of your bones. Both your cancer and your therapy may put them at risk. Metastatic prostate cancer eventually spreads to pelvis, hips, spine and other skeletal structures, leading to potential fractures and significant pain. In addition, hormone or androgen-deprivation therapy can cause bones to lose three to four percent of their mineral density, making them further prone to breaks. (The effect is similar to osteoporosis in postmenopausal women.)

Treatment for Bone Metastases

The primary goal of any prostate cancer treatment is to slow or even prevent the spread of cancerous cells throughout your body, especially to your bones. If those cells have already affected your skeletal structures, however, the additional goal is to alleviate pain and further complications. Although treatment for your disease may help with both challenges, you may need additional therapy to target problems created by bone metastases.

Your doctor may choose from various drugs:

- *Bisphosphonates (zoledronic acid,* referred to as Zometa). By slowing production of *osteoclasts,* cells that break down the hard mineral structure of bone, bisphosphonates strengthen bone and even delay fractures related to prostate cancer metastases. Osteoclasts ordinarily work in tandem with osteoblasts, cells that secrete new bone. Both are part of the normal bone-rebuilding and remodeling process, but in prostate cancer they become overactive, causing weakening and other problems for skeletal areas targeted by cancerous cells. Zometa, the only FDA-approved bisphosphonate for prostate cancer metastases, slows that process. It's administered intravenously, usually once every three or four weeks.

- *Denosumab* (Prolia, Xgeva). Like bisphosphonates, these drugs block osteoclasts, but in a slightly different way. By interfering with a protein necessary to activate osteoclasts (or the immature cells that become osteoclasts), these manufactured antibodies stop the bone-tissue-removing cells from reaching and damaging skeletal structures. In men whose cancer has already spread to the bone, denosumab can prevent or delay fractures. In men with no obvious signs of metastases but rising PSA despite hormone therapy, denosumab may slow cancer's spread. In either case, the drug is injected under the skin. Whether you take Zometa, Prolia, or Xgeva, your doctor will likely prescribe calcium and vitamin D supplements to restore depleted calcium.

- *Radiopharmaceuticals: Strontium-89* (Metastron), Samarium-153 (Quadramet), Radium-223 (Xofigo).Radiopharmaceuticals work by sending radioactive materials, called *radioisotopes,* to cancerous areas of the body. Metastron and Quadramet specifically target metastases of the bone. Injected intravenously into an arm vein, these drugs eventually collect in diseased sites. There they give off radiation particles that kill cancerous cells while easing the pain caused by a metastasis. Because radiopharmaceuticals travel throughout your skeletal and blood systems, they're particularly helpful if your cancer has spread to many bones. Though external beam radiation may be used as well for the most painful sites, radiopharmaceuticals can work alone to offer relief.

6   Chemotherapy

The role of chemotherapy in prostate cancer treatment is growing as new drugs come on the scene. More and more, oncologists integrate chemotherapy into treatment plans for men with advanced or late-stage prostate cancer—extending not just lives but quality of life as well. Though chemotherapy is not a cure, it can slow the growth and spread of cancerous cells while controlling symptoms.

What Is Chemotherapy?

Chemotherapy agents are potent chemicals designed to kill cancer cells throughout the body. These drugs work in various ways. Some prevent *angiogenesis,* the growth of new blood vessels through which cancer can spread. Others arrest cancer cells in different phases of their growth cycles. There are drugs that restore *apoptosis*—the normal cell death process, which cancer cells resist—while others attack DNA within cancer-cell genes to prevent cell growth and reproduction.

Historically, chemotherapy has had limited usefulness in treating prostate cancer. Because prostate cancer is slow growing, while chemotherapeutic agents work best on fast-growing cells, chemotherapy isn't practical for early-stage disease. In addition, chemotherapy drugs travel through the body, destroying healthy and malignant cells alike and producing undesirable side effects. In prostate cancer, the issue has always been, "Do the questionable or limited benefits outweigh the discomfort?"

Today, new and more effective chemotherapeutic agents—along with better medications to deal with side effects, and more accurate ways to measure how well an agent works—are making chemotherapy more appealing. In particular, it is good option for one type of cancer: hormone-insensitive late-stage disease.

When Is Chemotherapy Recommended?

Chemotherapy is a treatment option for a diagnosis of metastatic castration-resistant prostate cancer, the most challenging form of advanced prostate cancer. Doctors typically use chemotherapy only when significant symptoms (such as bone pain and urinary issues) and CT-scan confirmation leave no doubt that cancer is spreading.

Chemotherapy Drugs for Advanced Prostate Cancer

When chemotherapy is indicated, oncologists prescribe *docetaxel* (Taxotere), in the class of anticancer drugs called *taxoids*. This drug prevents cancer-cell division by interfering with particles called *microtubules* in the DNA or internal structure of the cell. With microtubules out of commission, the cell dies.

Because of its effectiveness, Taxotere has overtaken older chemotherapy agents as a first-line defense for mCRPC. If Taxotere fails to achieve the desired result, doctors may choose to forgo additional chemotherapy in favor of secondary hormone manipulations (described in chapter 5) or continue with another chemotherapeutic agent.

Cabazitaxel (Jevtana) is next to Taxotere in usefulness. Also a taxoid, it works like Taxotere and is administered in the same way: intravenously for one hour every three weeks. The oral steroid Prednisone is prescribed to deter allergic reactions and side effects.

Less common than the newer drug Jevtana, *mitoxantrone* or *estramustine phosphate* may also be tried.

- *Mitoxantrone* (Novantrone) is from a group anticancer drugs referred to as *anthracyclines*. Novantrone kills cancer cells by damaging their genes, thus interfering with reproduction. As with Taxetore and Jevtana, Novantrone is given intravenously every three weeks with oral Prednisone.

- *Estramustine phosphate* (Emcyte) slows or stops the growth of prostate cancer in two ways: It damages cancer cells so they can't divide and it increases production of the hormone estrogen, which impedes testosterone. Emcyte is taken orally, one capsule three or four times a day *without* Prednisone.

Discontinuing Chemotherapy or Using a Different Drug

In choosing to continue or change therapy, oncologists generally consider three factors:

- *Is the patient handling the chemotherapy well?* Doctors monitor patients' side effects and overall condition, determining whether the patients remain well enough to tolerate and benefit from the drugs.

- *Is the chemotherapy working?* The doctor examines various markers—such as a reduction in pain or CT/PET scan evidence of improvement—as indications of the therapy's effectiveness.

- *Are there major adverse events after chemotherapy?* If the medication seems to cause severe side effects, such as liver toxicity or a dramatic drop in white blood cells, patient and oncologist may decide to discontinue chemotherapy. At that point, the optimal choice may be pain medication to keep the patient comfortable.

Preparing for Chemotherapy

Before beginning chemotherapy, doctors order blood tests, X-rays and other imaging studies, and biopsies. These tests help the doctor locate metastases and determine whether the patient is a good candidate for chemotherapy. Patients in satisfactory health when chemotherapy begins are less likely than others to experience troublesome side effects.

Necessary dental work should be completed at least two weeks before treatments start. Having dental work during the course of chemotherapy is risky, since chemotherapy patients are especially vulnerable to infection and mouth sores. (As mentioned earlier, chemotherapy kills healthy fast-growing cells such as those in the lining of the mouth.)

Days or weeks before surgery, doctors may start patients on antinausea drugs and advise them to stay well hydrated and to avoid spicy and fatty foods. Food and fluids are generally off limits for at least two hours before a chemotherapy treatment.

Delivery of Chemotherapy

Except for drugs taken orally (by mouth, such as Emcyte capsules three or four times a day), chemotherapy is given in cycles—a treatment followed by a recovery period before the next treatment and recovery period.

Why are treatments given in cycles? Chemotherapy kills cancer cells that are rapidly dividing but doesn't affect those that are at rest. Repeated cycles improve the odds of finding and destroying cancer cells when they are in the reproduction phase. Time off between treatments allows normal tissues to recover. Chemotherapy may be administered once a week, but once every three weeks is usual.

How many cycles do patients undergo? For advanced prostate cancer, chemotherapy may continue as long as it is working and side effects are well tolerated.

Oral chemotherapy can usually be done at home. Chemotherapy in liquid form, by injection or IV drip

Chemotherapy Agents for Prostate Cancer
• *Docetaxel* (Taxotere)
• *Cabazitaxel* (Jevtana)
• *Mitoxantrone* (Novantrone)
• *Estramustine phosphate* (Emcyt)
• *Doxorubicin* (Adriamycin)
• *Etoposide* (VP-16)
• *Vinblastine* (Velban)
• *Paclitaxel* (Taxol)
• *Carboplatin* (Paraplatin)
• *Vinorelbine* (Navelbine)

(infusion) through a catheter or port, typically takes place in a clinic or hospital. Each treatment may take a few minutes to several hours, depending on the drug, the dose, and the delivery method. Some doctors admit chemotherapy patients to the hospital for overnight observation after the first treatment.

Comparatively frequent low doses tend to be more comfortable for patients, and possibly more effective, than fewer, larger doses. Slow-growing prostate cancer cells require longer exposure to cancer-fighting chemicals than do fast-growing cells. With daily oral doses or frequent injections, overall exposure is greater and side effects are reduced.

What is a PICC Line?

One way of giving frequent low doses at an effective level is through a *peripherally inserted central catheter (PICC) line.* Similar to an IV, a PICC line is a long, thin, flexible plastic tube through which medication is delivered and blood samples can be drawn. The PICC remains painlessly in place throughout the course of treatment so there's no need to hunt for a vein and insert a new needle at every treatment.

After applying a local anesthetic, a doctor or specially trained nurse inserts the PICC line, usually in the upper arm. The tube is carefully threaded through the body into a large vein next to the heart where blood flow quickly distributes medication throughout the body. Patients need only ensure that the insertion site remain covered, clean, and dry while the PICC line is in place.

As a bonus, the PICC greatly reduces the risk of *extravasation injury,* damage that occurs around the injection site when chemotherapy drugs leak into nearby tissues. If extravasation injury does occur, the doctor can prescribe a medicinal cream to rub onto the injured area.

Risks, Complications, and Side Effects of Chemotherapy

Chemotherapy's action is *systemic,* meaning that it affects the entire body. Though chemotherapy drugs can attack both normal and malignant cells anywhere in the body, the drugs target primarily fast-growing or rapidly dividing cells, such as those in bone marrow, hair follicles, and the reproductive and digestive systems—accounting for potential hair loss and nausea. Side effects differ with particular drugs and combinations. Medications and other strategies are available to lessen or eliminate these side effects.

Potential side effects can seem overwhelming. Keep in mind:

- Not everyone experiences every side effect.
- Side effects usually resolve when the body has a chance to recover after chemotherapy.
- There are a number of chemotherapy drugs to choose from, so if one is particularly troublesome, another may be better tolerated.
- Uncomfortable side effects can be alleviated with prescription drugs, over-the-counter products, lifestyle adjustments, and other strategies. It's important to mention side effects to the oncologist as soon as they occur so they can be quickly dealt with.

Fatigue

One of the most common side effects of chemotherapy is fatigue, often brought on by a low red blood cell count (anemia). Red blood cells deliver oxygen throughout the body. Inadequate oxygen supplies in tissues and organs cause fatigue. Severe anemia during chemotherapy can be treated with a blood transfusion or a medication that stimulates production of red blood cells.

For some patients, fatigue occurs around the time of a treatment. Others feel fatigued during the entire course of therapy or beyond, after chemotherapy has ended. It can take weeks for energy to return to normal. For active patients, fatigue can be a source of frustration, even depression. It's best to stay positive and remember that the fatigue is temporary.

Here are a few tips for coping with fatigue:

- Limit activities; do only those things that are most important.
- Take several short naps or breaks during the day.

- Try taking short walks or exercising lightly.
- Maintain good nutrition; try to eat a well-balanced diet.
- Ask for help.

Digestive Tract Side Effects

Chemotherapy can cause a variety of side effects throughout the digestive tract. Nausea, vomiting, constipation, diarrhea, loss of appetite, and mouth and throat sores can afflict patients undergoing chemotherapy. Not everyone experiences all these side effects, which can vary with the type of drug, the dose, and the frequency and duration of chemotherapy.

Irritation of the stomach and intestinal lining can cause diarrhea and abdominal cramping lasting several hours to several days. With severe diarrhea there is a risk of dehydration and loss of nutrients. Patients may be hospitalized for intravenous fluid replacement.

To prevent digestive problems or ease their severity:

- Drink at least six to eight glasses of water daily.
- Avoid high-fiber, greasy, rich, and spicy foods; any food high in sugar; caffeine drinks; and alcohol.
- Eat small amounts of solid food frequently throughout the day.
- Eat and drink slowly; chew foods well.
- Suck on ice cubes, mints, or ginger candies (unless prevented by mouth sores).

Many adults are lactose intolerant; their bodies have stopped making the lactase enzyme needed to digest milk sugar (lactose). For these people, milk and milk products can cause diarrhea or constipation, especially during chemotherapy. Try yogurt or buttermilk, which contain beneficial bacteria that basically predigest the lactose for you.

Check with your doctor before using over-the-counter products such as Imodium-AD for diarrhea or milk of magnesia for constipation. There are prescription drugs available for these conditions.

Diarrhea, vomiting, and inability to eat can be dangerous, causing you to become malnourished or dehydrated. It's important to tell your doctor if you're experiencing any of these symptoms. Don't assume they're just part of the treatment process.

Mouth Sores

Mouth and throat sores can be aggravated both by a low white-blood-cell count and by chemotherapy's effects on your digestive system. Mouth sores *(stomatitis)* are less common with chemotherapy for prostate cancer than for other cancers, but they can arise with any chemotherapy, subsiding when treatments come to an end.

These sores emerge as painful lesions or ulcers on the lips, in the mouth, on the gums, and inside the throat. More than uncomfortable, mouth sores may make eating and drinking difficult, and dehydration can result. Infection is also a possibility.

If you develop mouth sores, ask your doctor about medication to treat them. Here are other ways to deal with mouth sores:

- If possible, have your teeth cleaned and dental work completed before starting chemotherapy.
- Brush and floss your teeth often, using a soft-bristle brush to avoid irritating gums.
- Avoid mouthwashes that contain alcohol. Some doctors recommend rinsing your mouth with a

mild salt-water solution, while others claim that salt can worsen mouth sores.

- Stay hydrated by drinking plenty of water.
- Suck on ice chips; they may be soothing.
- Eat soft foods, such as baby food, cooled oatmeal, mashed vegetables, yogurt, ice cream, milk shakes, and smoothies. Avoid hard, crunchy foods and those with high acid content (tomatoes, citrus fruits), a lot of salt or spices, and caffeine. Don't smoke or chew tobacco.
- Try this homemade gargle: Mix one-half teaspoon of salt and one teaspoon of baking soda in one quart of water, and gargle every four hours.

Neuropathy

Chemotherapy can cause *neuropathy,* a form of nerve damage manifesting in pain, numbness, or tingling sensations in various parts of the body. Severity depends on how much of the chemotherapy agent you received and how quickly it was administered. It's essential to report neuropathy symptoms to your oncologist right away so that he or she can adjust or suspend treatment.

Commonly, neuropathy occurs in the hands and feet. In the hands, it may interfere with activities such as buttoning a shirt, typing, writing, or playing a musical instrument. Neuropathy in the mouth, throat, or chest can show up as abnormal tongue sensations, a choking sensation, or a feeling of pressure on your chest.

Neuropathy may be either acute or chronic. Acute neuropathy goes away within days after a chemotherapy treatment, while chronic neuropathy can persist for weeks to months. Symptoms may be constant, or they may come and go. The chronic form of neuropathy can become irreversible if treatment continues, so the oncologist may reduce the chemotherapy dose or stop the treatment altogether.

Folic acid, one of the B vitamins, has been shown in numerous studies to be effective against chemotherapy-induced neuropathy. Medications are also available to alleviate neuropathy pain.

Infections

Chemotherapy can damage the bone marrow, where blood cells originate. Up to 70 percent of circulating white blood cells are *neutrophils,* which destroy bacteria in the blood. A neutrophil deficiency, called *neutropenia,* as well as a low white-blood-cell count in general, signifies a compromised immune system. Since the immune system wards off disease, its impairment leaves an opening for infections of the blood, urinary tract, skin, and other sites, and for pneumonia.

Be alert for signs of infection—fever over 100 degrees Fahrenheit, shaking, chills, or sweats; coughing up dark or bloody sputum; pain or burning with urination; and pain or redness around cuts. If you feel an infection coming on, notify your doctor immediately. Infections can be effectively treated with antibiotics.

To reduce your risk of infection, take these precautions:

- Wash your hands often during the day, especially after using the bathroom.
- Avoid anyone who has a cold, flu, measles, or chicken pox.
- Stay away from children who have recently received vaccinations.
- Clean cuts and scrapes right away.

- Wear gloves when gardening or cleaning up after pets or children.
- Use a soft toothbrush that won't hurt your gums.
- Clean yourself thoroughly after each bowel movement; if the area around your anus becomes irritated or if you have hemorrhoids, notify your doctor.

Impaired Blood Clotting

Chemotherapy can also cause a condition called *thrombocytopenia,* indicated by a low blood platelet count. Platelets are blood cells that help with clotting. Mild thrombocytopenia may produce no symptoms. A severe deficiency of platelets may show up in a purplish rash on the hands and feet or easy bruising, both of which signify bleeding under the skin. Spontaneous nosebleeds may occur. In serious cases, there can be internal bleeding.

There are no medications for this condition, and a physician will usually delay or suspend chemotherapy when a patient's blood platelet count is low. This break in treatment gives the platelet count time to rise on its own. If the platelet count drops dangerously, however, a blood platelet transfusion may be needed to avoid bleeding complications.

Once the course of chemotherapy has ended, low blood counts are treatable and reversible. Throughout your treatment, your doctor will monitor your blood counts.

Hair and Nail Changes

There are chemotherapy patients who never have problems with their hair or nails. Most experience at least some changes, however.

As chemotherapy destroys cancer cells, it also destroys the rapidly reproducing cells responsible for hair and nail growth. Once chemotherapy is completed, these cells usually recover and hair and nails go back to normal. Often, the new hair growth is a slightly different color or texture than it was before chemotherapy, but the change is usually temporary. Although hair loss can occur anywhere on the body, it is mainly confined to the head.

It usually takes a few weeks for the hair to start thinning. It becomes brittle, eventually breaking off near the roots or falling out altogether. Some patients wear hats, scarves, or wigs to cover their heads and stay warm. Others decide to shave off all their hair at this point, in part because wigs stay on better and are more comfortable on a bald scalp. You may simply choose to go bald and enjoy the temporary freedom from washing and cutting your hair. Do wear a cap and sunscreen outdoors to prevent sunburn.

Your insurance may cover the cost of a wig or hair prosthesis. The latter is basically a wig that is custom designed and fitted so it looks natural.

At this time, little can be done to prevent chemotherapy-induced hair loss—not a dangerous side effect but sometimes a distressing one. There are no drugs, food supplements, or hair treatment products that can prevent it, despite the claims that appear on the Internet and in magazine ads. Your doctor and your support group can suggest ways to cope with hair loss. In general:

- Use mild shampoos.
- Use a soft hairbrush.
- Use low heat on your hair dryer.
- Don't dye your hair.
- Protect your scalp from the sun with a hat or sunscreen.

Fingernails and toenails won't fall off, but white bands might appear on them and they may also change color. Keeping them short and filed smooth not only will improve their appearance, it will keep you from accidentally tearing a nail or giving yourself a scratch.

Skin Changes

During chemotherapy, your skin may be itchy and dry. You'll probably be susceptible to sunburn, and you might develop a rash, sores, or blisters—all normal to a degree. Be sure to let your doctor know if these conditions are severe, however, because skin abnormalities can signal an allergic reaction to chemotherapy drugs. To prevent infection, immediately call your doctor's attention to any open sores.

If your skin is flaking, your bedding harbors dead skin and bacteria, so change your sheets often. Take warm but not hot showers and baths. Baking soda in your bath water can soothe itching. Ask your doctor about taking vitamin E or zinc supplements. Your doctor might also recommend skin products containing aloe vera or oatmeal (such as Alpha Keri). Use mild skin cleansers, shampoos, and laundry products (such as Dreft and Ivory Snow, which are gentle enough for babies' sensitive skin). Wear sunscreen, at least 15 SPF, any time you go outdoors. Drink plenty of fluids to hydrate your skin, and avoid extremes of heat or cold.

Nervous System Changes

Some chemotherapy drugs can damage the nervous system and may have an effect on brain functions. Tell your doctor immediately about symptoms such as headache, confusion, depression, fever, numbness or tingling in the extremities, dry mouth, vision problems, and· ringing in the ears. Prescription medication may prevent many of these problems.

Doctors sometimes prescribe antidepressants for chemotherapy-related depression and other symptoms. Anticonvulsants can alleviate pain that stems from nervous system damage. Increasingly, doctors are recommending acupuncture and acupressure, which may effectively relieve pain for many patients not helped by drugs.

Impairments referred to as "brain fog" are usually mild but can be frustrating. You might feel confused, have problems concentrating, or have trouble finding the word you want to use to express yourself.

This side effect may linger from months to years. The severity of it depends on how much chemotherapy was given and for how long. If you find yourself coping with memory and thinking impairments, here are steps you can take:

- Keep a notepad handy to jot down reminders to yourself.
- Keep a calendar nearby for scheduling appointments and events.
- Get plenty of rest.
- Ask for support from family members and friends.

Some patients report that exercise, music therapy, art, or reading helps them deal with memory and thinking impairments.

Kidney and Liver Damage

A few chemotherapy drugs may cause liver or kidney damage, which can sometimes be prevented with prescription drugs. Regular blood tests monitor kidney and liver function. If damage is suspected, another chemotherapy drug may be used.

After Chemotherapy

After you complete your chemotherapy, your medical oncologist will want to see you for follow-up examinations. As part of the follow-up, you'll have blood tests, X-rays, and scans. Your oncologist will also want to monitor any side effects that are likely to linger. Report all side effects and any other problems during your follow-up visits.

7 Life after Prostate Cancer

If you're recovering from prostate cancer treatment or you're having hormone therapy, your body has changed, and may continue to change, in ways you might find confusing, embarrassing, even depressing. Take heart. There's help for you—medical, spiritual, and emotional—though for many men, the most difficult thing is to ask for it.

Think of all the *giving* you've done in your life—to family, friends, your job, perhaps your place of worship—and allow yourself to *take* for a change. Take advantage of the many resources that are available to you from organizations, medical professionals, family, friends, books and tapes, pastors, and counselors. Take some time for yourself and your loved ones. Take time to do the things you've always wanted to do. Be kind to yourself. Pamper yourself. Many men report that they enjoy life more because they learned so much about living life and enjoying it to the fullest.

Coping Emotionally
Support Groups

Some of the most powerful support available comes from men like you—prostate cancer survivors who are grateful to be alive. These men gather in community centers and hospital meeting rooms, or in online discussion groups, to share their stories, draw strength from each other, and learn about prostate cancer treatment advances. More than anyone else, they know what you've been through and what you're facing. They can recommend physicians and therapists, books and videos, organizations and other resources. With their help you can learn to talk about your illness and the effect it's having on your life.

There's at least one more good reason to get involved with a support group. Studies have consistently shown that cancer patients in strong support groups live longer. Strong is a key word here. Most support groups are upbeat and encouraging. A few are dominated by pessimists, naysayers, or people who just won't stop talking. If you find yourself in one of these, seek out another one. The last thing you need is to surround yourself with gloom and doom, especially when there's so much to feel good about.

How do you find a support group? First, ask your urologist. Actually, you probably won't even have to ask. Physicians know the value of such support and routinely steer their patients toward relevant support groups. You can also get local meeting information online or by calling or writing the American Cancer Society or the prostate cancer support organizations Man to Man and Us Too! For details on these and other sources of information and support, see the Resources section in the back of this book.

Spiritual Resources

Some men gain a sense of well-being in prayer or fellowship groups, yoga classes, and meditation gatherings. Through the ages, people have relied on prayer, pastoral counseling, and close-knit religious communities to help them through illness and other difficulties. Many members of the clergy in nearly every denomination have received training in pastoral counseling. A growing number of physicians actively recommend these spiritual resources to their patients, not only because of their own faith experiences but also because of new research that validates the role of prayer and church attendance in healing and prolonging life.

Help for Depression

It's not uncommon for men to get depressed, anxious, or both when their prostate cancer is diagnosed. You might have been devastated when you found out you had prostate cancer and thrilled when you learned about curative treatment options. Maybe you were nervous before surgery or radiation but depressed in the aftermath when your energy flagged and your bowels didn't work right. Perhaps you were anxious when you wondered if that ache or that slightly elevated PSA meant your cancer had returned.

Talk to your doctor right away. Don't delay getting help for depression or anxiety. A cheerful outlook is your best friend. With medication, counseling, or a combination of the two, you can find the tools that are so important right now to take care of yourself, stay informed, and participate fully and joyfully in life.

Talk to Your Partner

If you have a mate, hopefully you have emotional support and can share your fears and joys. Perhaps you have a close friend or relative you can count on to be there for you. Maybe you're a person who has held things in all your life. Perhaps you've thought that being "strong" meant dealing with your problems on your own. Maybe it's time to let down your defenses and stop being a hero.

Please realize that your prostate cancer affects those who love you almost as much as it affects you, even if you don't talk about it openly. Couples who go through big changes together, keeping the lines of communication open, usually emerge stronger and closer than they were before. This is an opportunity for your relationship to grow.

Take your spouse or partner with you to doctors' appointments and support group meetings. Share your hopes and fears. You're entitled to them. Discuss treatment options, side effects, the possibility of impotence or incontinence, and the information you gather. Two heads really are better than one when you're trying to solve a problem, make a decision, or overcome anxiety.

Your Children, Family Members, Friends, and Coworkers

What should you tell the kids? Many counselors recommend a balance between honesty and reassurance, depending on your children's ages, and advise against trying to protect them by keeping them in the dark. Grown children are likely to be hurt if they're deprived of a chance to help and support their dad, and even very young children know and become anxious when something disquieting is going on.

What you say to other people depends on your relationship with them and their need to know. Don't worry that you're burdening people when you tell them about your illness. Most people are eager to help when they can, even if it's just by listening. On the other hand, your fellow cocktail party guests would probably prefer not to hear the toe-curling details of your orchiectomy or brachytherapy procedure.

When people ask how they can help, tell them. Do you need transportation to the doctor's office or the hospital? Do you just want someone to listen? Let them know! If they genuinely care about you, you'll be doing them a favor by letting them contribute to your well-being.

Your Doctor Can Help

Your doctor and his or her staff can give you information, referrals, and encouragement. Be assured that your urologist and probably your primary care doctor have heard every embarrassing question in the book, from "What kind of undergarment is best for leakage?" to "What kind of penile implant is most 'natural' and safest?" If you're not completely honest with your doctor, you risk losing access to a drug or procedure that could make your life a lot more enjoyable.

Coping with Incontinence

Some degree of incontinence is likely after radical prostatectomy or radiation therapy. It's almost always temporary, though in some cases it can be a problem for years. After radiation therapy, incontinence may get worse over time because radiation-damaged cells can't repair themselves as other cells do.

Bladder control in healthy men depends on the *urinary sphincter* muscles at the bladder neck and below the bladder around the urethra. Prostate surgery or radiation can damage or weaken these muscles so that they can no longer keep urine from leaking out of the bladder.

Prostate cancer treatment usually causes *stress urinary incontinence,* involuntary leaking of urine when you cough, sneeze, laugh, or get up out of a chair. After radical prostatectomy, more than 95 percent of patients regain continence, many fairly quickly, though it can take as long as three years. Less common with prostate cancer are *urge incontinence,* when you can't get to the bathroom in time, and *overflow incontinence,* when normal urine flow is blocked and the bladder is always full.

Medications for Incontinence

Depending on the type of incontinence you have, your doctor might prescribe simple decongestants, antidepressants, or other drugs to help you regain urinary retention. Drugs are usually the first line of defense in treating incontinence.

Decongestants, which may tighten the urethral muscles, are often prescribed for stress incontinence. These drugs are also called *alpha-adrenergic agonists* and contain ingredients such as ephedrine and pseudoephedrine that are found in nonprescription decongestants and appetite suppressants. If you have high blood pressure, heart disease, diabetes, hyperthyroidism, or glaucoma, you should not take alpha-adrenergic agonists.

For urge incontinence, *anticholinergic agents,* normally used to treat Parkinson's disease, can help by delaying the urge to urinate and allowing the bladder to hold more urine. Patients have complained about anticholinergic agents' unpleasant side effects—dry eyes and mouth, constipation, and rapid heartbeat—but newer versions of these drugs may be much easier to tolerate.

Tricyclic antidepressants such as *imipramine* (Tofranil) and *amitriptyline* (Elavil) can help control stress incontinence by tightening the bladder neck muscles. They are not prescribed for people with heart disease and can cause a host of side effects, from dizziness and sweating to dry mouth, headache, constipation, and ringing in the ears. Possible, though uncommon, are more serious side effects, including seizures, heart attack, high blood pressure, and allergic reactions. These drugs can also do their job too well, causing urinary retention.

Exercises for Incontinence

One of the best and easiest ways, and certainly the cheapest way, to overcome or diminish the incontinence problem is with *Kegel exercises,* also called *pelvic floor exercises.* These are so simple you can do them almost anywhere. Simply tighten your pelvic muscles, keep them tight for about ten seconds, and then release.

You use your pelvic muscles many times a day. They're the muscles you tighten to keep from urinating before you can get to the bathroom. To practice, try stopping the urine stream after you've begun urinating. Some doctors tell their prostate cancer patients to do Kegels for five minutes twenty or so times each day, starting even before treatment. After treatment, keep up this regimen until you're no longer troubled with incontinence.

Your doctor may refer you to physical therapy for help rehabilitating your pelvic muscles. You might not think Kegel exercises would be difficult to master, but it's surprisingly easy to do them wrong. It's important to tighten only the pelvic muscles, not the buttocks or the abdominal or thigh muscles. Some physical therapists use biofeedback to teach the proper way to do Kegel exercises.

Biofeedback to reinforce pelvic floor exercises is easy and painless. You'll be hooked up to a machine that lights up or gives another clear signal when you do the exercise correctly. As you repeatedly try to stimulate the signal, you get better and better at the exercise until it becomes second nature.

The Male Sling

This new procedure, in which a strip of abdominal or synthetic tissue is surgically placed in the pelvis to compress the urethra, can usually be done on an outpatient basis in less than half an hour. It requires only a two-inch incision between the scrotum and the rectum. The male sling is not yet widely available, but early studies have shown improvement in 80 percent of the men treated. Many doctors predict that the male sling will become the treatment of choice for male urinary incontinence.

The Condom Catheter

A condom catheter is a simple device that drains leaked urine from the penis. The condom, usually latex, is attached to the penis with adhesive. A plastic tube connects the condom catheter to a bag taped to the leg. The urine stays in the attached leg bag until it is emptied.

If you are allergic to latex, the condom catheter probably isn't for you. Many doctors recommend against the device for other reasons as well. Besides being a crutch that can prevent men from working to regain urinary control, the condom catheter may contribute to urinary tract infections and other problems. If you want to use the condom catheter, do so only under your doctor's supervision and only for brief outings, since the bag must be emptied every thirty minutes.

Penile Clamp

An external penile clamp (called a *Cunningham clamp*) can be effective in controlling incontinence. Worn over the penis, the clamp exerts pressure on the urethra, stopping leakage. When used as prescribed, the clamp is safe and convenient. This inexpensive device is probably available from your urologist.

Artificial Urinary Sphincter

If you have lingering incontinence, consider an artificial urinary sphincter, which involves a simple surgical procedure done on an outpatient basis or with an overnight hospital stay. The surgeon places a small balloon in your lower abdomen, an inflatable cuff around the urethra, and a pump in the scrotum.

When the cuff contains fluid it compresses the urethra so that urine can't escape. When you want to urinate, you squeeze the pump a few times. Activating the pump causes the fluid to flow from the cuff to the balloon. After you urinate, the fluid will flow back into the cuff.

The procedure is successful up to 90 percent of the time and carries minimal risk. As with any minor surgery, there's a slight chance of bleeding or infection. Rare complications can include urinary retention and malfunction or breakage of the device. The artificial sphincter is not a good option for older men, for men who have had radiation therapy, or for those who have vascular disease.

Collagen Injections

Collagen is a natural protein that's commonly used in cosmetic procedures to plump up facial skin and diminish fine lines and wrinkles. The same principle applies in this simple outpatient procedure; when collagen is injected into the tissues around the bladder neck, they swell to prevent urine leakage out of the bladder. Only men with mild incontinence benefit from collagen injections, which have to be repeated—two or three times initially and again if the leakage comes back. The procedure can remain effective for mere months to many years, though the average is a few years.

Your doctor will do a skin test to make sure you're not allergic to the collagen, which is derived from cattle. This is a very important precaution, as an allergic reaction could be life threatening. If you've had a radical prostatectomy followed by radiation therapy, collagen injections will not work for you; the injections can't "bulk up" the radiation-treated bladder neck.

Incontinence Undergarments

In every drugstore you'll find shelves covered with a great variety of disposable pads and underpants for adults with incontinence. Some are made specifically for men. They're very useful, even necessary, immediately after a radical prostatectomy. You probably don't relish the idea of prowling the store aisles looking for the perfect incontinence product, but reassure yourself that it's just a short-term measure and keep doing your Kegels. Ask your doctor which product he or she recommends. Change your pad or undergarment often to avoid odor and chafing.

Coping with Impotence

Every medical treatment for prostate cancer carries a risk of temporary or permanent impotence. It's impossible to know before treatment which men will become impotent and for how long. Even among men in their forties who have the nerve-sparing radical prostatectomy, with both neurovascular bundles preserved, and who had good erections before surgery, 10 percent remain impotent afterward.

Normally, when you start to get an erection, blood flows into the chambers in the penis. It is the blood in these chambers that keeps the penis erect. While you're aroused, the blood vessels are sealed off and the blood can't flow back out. This natural process may not work well, or at all, after prostate cancer treatment.

During prostate surgery or radiation, blood vessels and nerve pathways to the penis are damaged to a greater or lesser extent, and impotence occurs. Hormone therapy causes impotence in an entirely different way, by eliminating testosterone, the hormone that governs male sexuality, from the body. During hormone therapy for prostate cancer—essentially chemical castration—men not only become impotent, they lose interest in sex. Potency may return when treatment stops. This is not the case with orchiectomy, in which the source of nearly all the body's testosterone is surgically removed. Surgical castration produces permanent impotence and loss of sex drive.

Some men hope to be spared the problem of impotence by delaying treatment as long as possible or forgoing it altogether. The fact is, impotence can occur without treatment. In fact, impotence is as much a complication of the disease as it is of the treatment.

With or without prostate cancer, 25 percent of men will be impotent by age 65. Impotence can be a result of diabetes, hypertension, and other disorders, as well as medications, alcohol, smoking, and psychological conditions.

Fortunately, a great deal can be done to help men who have some degree of impotence. Please keep in mind that the word *impotence* refers only to the inability to have an erection. Other facets of sexual activity—libido (sexual desire), ejaculation, and orgasm—are separate. If you are impotent, you can usually continue to enjoy sex and have orgasms.

Better than any device or procedure to restore erections are trust and communication between you and your partner. Be willing to talk openly and to experiment with techniques you both find enjoyable, whether or not they produce an erection.

Drugs for Impotence

The availability of Viagra, Levitra, and Cialis has been a boon to prostate cancer patients and other men with impotence or erectile dysfunction. These drugs, called *PDE-*

5 inhibitors, work by blocking an enzyme, *phosphodies-terase type 5,* found in penile tissues. When the enzyme is blocked, the smooth muscles of the penis can relax to allow blood to flow in.

PDE-5 inhibitors work well for a majority of men. Your doctor may tell you to start taking one of these drugs before your treatment, or afterward just prior to resuming intercourse.

Viagra, Levitra, and Cialis are not aphrodisiacs. They won't help you become aroused. You have to provide the libido; the drug can help supply the erection.

Most men tolerate PDE-5 inhibitors well, but there are some men who should never take them. If you have coronary artery disease, get clearance from your cardiologist before using the drug. If you're taking medicine containing nitrates (such as nitroglycerine or isosorbides), PDE-5 inhibitors are not for you. The combination can cause a dangerous drop in blood pressure. Side effects, though uncommon, can include headache, flushing, indigestion, runny nose, diarrhea, dizziness, and a temporary blue haze or other eyesight disturbance.

Penile Injections

Less unpleasant than they sound, penile injections are actually an easy, painless, and effective way to achieve a normal erection. Using a small syringe with a very fine needle, you'll inject a *vasodilator,* a drug that widens blood vessels, into the penis shaft. The vasodilator opens the blood vessels and relaxes the smooth muscles of the penis. Within ten to twenty minutes, both chambers fill with blood, giving you an erection that lasts thirty minutes to two hours.

If you have heart disease, ask your doctor if vasodilators are safe for you. This technique won't work for you if

Penile Pump

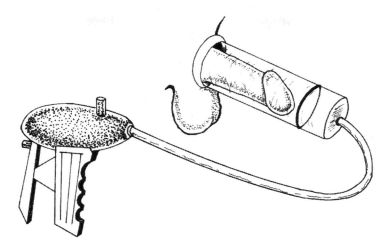

A penile pump is used externally to make blood flow into the shaft and tip of the penis, causing an erection.

for some reason you're unable to give yourself the injection, whether because of squeamishness, poor eyesight, or poor coordination.

It's important that you take the lowest effective dose possible. If the dose is too high, you could have a prolonged erection that could actually become dangerous.

Other side effects can include very small blood clots, burning pain after the injection, damage to the urethra, and fibrous tissue buildup in the *corpora cavernosa.* Infection, if you've taken sanitary precautions, should never be a problem.

You've probably heard about men who use testosterone injections to restore sexual function. Be assured that no reputable doctor will prescribe testosterone for you if you are at risk or being treated for prostate cancer. Testosterone won't produce the desired effect and it could spur the growth of cancerous cells in your body.

Vacuum Erection Devices

A vacuum erection device is basically an airtight tube that you place over your lubricated penis. When you activate the attached pump, it creates a vacuum that draws blood into your penis. To keep the blood from flowing right back out, there's a rubber ring that slides off the tube and onto the base of the penis. These rings come in different sizes. If you have the correct size, it won't be uncomfortable.

Vacuum erection devices are safe and effective. You can use them as often as you like, but you must remove the ring after thirty minutes to restore healthy blood flow.

Penile Implants

There are several types of penile implants, or prostheses, all of which work well to produce erections in men who would otherwise be unable to have them. They are inserted into the penis surgically, under anesthetic, through a small incision in the scrotum. Some models have a reservoir, which is implanted in the abdomen, and a pump implanted in the scrotum. The procedure can be done on an outpatient basis or with an overnight stay in the hospital. All implants create a slight increase in penile diameter.

Some complex implants are inflatable and, in principle, much like an artificial sphincter. The surgeon implants a fluid reservoir and a cylinder in the penis. When you activate the device, it transfers fluid from the reservoir to the cylinder, creating an erection.

In general, the more sophisticated the device the more likely it is to malfunction, although all models are generally reliable. There are slight risks of infection, scarring, or damage to the two chambers that run the length of the penis.

Penile Implant

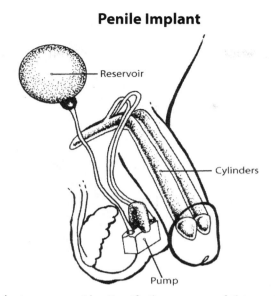

Penile implants are a consideration if other measures fail to produce erections. Long-term data shows penile implants to be highly effective and reliable.

Men often worry that penile implants made of silicone will cause problems similar to those of women who had silicone breast implants a few decades ago. This is simply not the case. In the few instances of the body's rejection, the device has simply been removed.

Penile implants are a consideration if other measures fail to produce erections. Long-term data show penile implants to be highly effective and reliable.

After Prostate Cancer: Follow-Up Care

You'll need to see your doctor regularly to have a PSA blood test and a urinalysis to check for blood in the urine. Your PSA should be 0.0 after surgery, although a PSA of 0.1 or 0.2 shouldn't alarm you, as lab tests have a slight margin of error. After radiation therapy, your PSA will drop slowly, ideally to below 0.5.

pect to see your doctor three or four times during the first year after treatment, two or three times a year for the next few years, and once or twice a year thereafter if things are going well. A slight rise in your PSA on one of these visits needn't mean trouble. Your doctor may repeat the test a few months later.

After your primary treatment for prostate cancer, your doctor might recommend a diet and exercise regimen to discourage the return of cancer and make you healthier and more energetic at the same time. A high-fiber, low-fat diet can prevent or improve many medical conditions. Ask your doctor to refer you to a nutritionist who can help you streamline a diet according to your preferences and needs.

If Cancer Recurs

Anyone who has had cancer knows what it's like to worry about a recurrence. For a while at least, every little symptom can set alarm bells ringing. You don't want to live every day in a state of heightened anxiety, but you're wise to be concerned and check with your doctor when your body sends you signals you don't understand. As is true with the initial diagnosis of prostate cancer, the earlier a recurrence is discovered, the better the chance of successfully managing the disease.

Your doctor will be alert to any PSA increase. If your PSA continues to rise, it probably means the cancer has returned. A rapid increase signals an aggressive cancer. This is by no means good news, but there are many avenues of treatment for men whose prostate cancer recurs. An issue that doctors still don't agree on is when to start salvage therapy–treatment after the primary treatment has failed.

Salvage Therapy

Many doctors will recommend salvage radiation treatments if cancer recurs after radical prostatectomy, possibly while your PSA is between 1.0 and 2.0. If your primary treatment was radiation (EBRT or brachytherapy), your doctor may want to start hormone therapy when your PSA is between 3.0 and 4.0. Hormone treatments probably won't get rid of your cancer altogether, but they can prolong your life and improve your quality of life for many years.

Performing a salvage prostatectomy after radiation is not unheard of, but it can be dangerous and difficult. Because of tissue damage, there's a good chance of injury to the rectal wall. The patient might require a permanent *colostomy,* a surgical procedure in which the large intestine is routed to an opening in the body through which fecal waste passes into an external bag. He might also be permanently incontinent.

Eventually, prostate cancer can spread through the lymph system, to the bones and elsewhere. Symptoms of metastatic cancer are many and varied—fatigue, weight loss, bone pain, loss of appetite, anemia, and others. With bone loss comes the risk of pathologic fractures, bones that break practically on their own, especially the weight-bearing bones of the hips and thighs.

Palliative Care

If the disease cannot be stopped, the purpose of treatment becomes palliative, intended to keep patients as comfortable as possible. Spot radiation, localized EBRT to painful bones, can shrink tumors and relieve pain for several weeks or months. Injections of radioactive materials target cancer in the bones and provide relief for up to six months. These injections can create a drop in blood production in the bone marrow, necessitating blood transfusions. For 48 hours after an injection, it's important to dispose of urine in the same way other radioactive materials are disposed of.

Spot radiation can also prevent spinal cord compression. This is a very serious condition that, if untreated, can lead to paralysis. Remedies include steroid drugs, surgical decompression, and orchiectomy.

There is no need for any man to be in continuous pain from prostate cancer. In the past, doctors and other health care professionals were afraid to overprescribe pain medication for fear of addiction or serious side effects. Patients have often cooperated with this reluctance by not asking for medication no matter how great their pain might be.

Today there's new awareness of the unnecessary suffering cancer patients have endured, and patients and their loved ones are being encouraged to make their needs known loud and clear. There is no such thing as pain that is unresponsive to medication. Painkillers range from mild (nonsteroidal anti-inflammatory drugs, or NSAIDs) to morphine strength, and anyone who is in great pain is entitled to take advantage of the many remedies available.

Other Approaches to Treatment

Nontraditional approaches can effectively supplement standard medical care. Biofeedback, meditation, relaxation techniques, hypnosis, acupuncture, and acupressure not only help patients relax and improve their outlook, they've earned the respect of the scientific community as well.

At any point in your treatment, speak up about every concern—pain or even mild discomfort, symptoms that alarm you, changes in the way your body functions. Don't assume that these problems just come with the territory. Scientists have spent years developing solutions for the very problems you may be having.

In Closing

The treatments available today for treating prostate cancer have saved the lives of many men. Clearly, the earlier a cancer is detected, the greater the chances for a cure. Although currently treatments are successful in many cases, new forms of treatment are always being developed and tested.

For example, one of the types of treatment being rigorously investigated is targeted focal therapy, which refers to several minimally invasive procedures that can destroy small, early-stage tumors while preserving healthy prostate tissue. These treatments, generally done on an outpatient basis, may eliminate cancer in men who would otherwise be considered for active surveillance or watchful waiting. In fact, some doctors refer to focal therapy as a "bridge" between active surveillance and aggressive treatment such as surgery or radiation. Focal therapy for the prostate has been called the "male version" of a breast-cancer lumpectomy.

Not all scientists are optimistic about focal therapy, however. Some object to using focal therapy as an alternative to active surveillance in low-risk patients, even for men who are anxious about their disease and request treatment. Such anxiety, say some experts, should be addressed with education and counseling, not unnecessary cancer treatment. Until persuasive long-term data on focal therapies becomes available, these treatments will remain controversial.

Diverse technologies are used in focal therapy; these technologies include the use of: lasers, freezing tissues, high-intensity heat waves, electrical currents, and nontoxic chemicals that enter a tumor and then kill cancer cells when the chemical is exposed to a certain type of light therapy.

There are risks with any medical procedure, especially if general anesthesia is required. However, compared to more aggressive forms of treatment, the focal therapies carry a lower risk of infection or bleeding, and there is little to no pain. Some procedures require the use of a urethral catheter for a few days or weeks because the swelling of tissues impairs urination.

Problems with urinary or erectile function, if any, are usually temporary according to the limited data available. In fact, because the focal therapies are still being studied in clinical trials and are not available as mainstream treatments, there are only a small number of doctors with expertise and experience in the procedures, and the unavailability of long-term studies to confirm safety and effectiveness.

Appendix

Simplified Summary of TNM Staging System
for Prostate Cancer

T = Tumor **N** = Nodes **M** = Metastases

Stage T1

Tumor is microscopic and confined to prostate but is undetectable by a digital rectal exam (DRE) or by ultrasound. Usually discovered by PSA tests or biopsies.

Stage T2

Tumor is confined to prostate and can be detected by DRE or ultrasound.

Stage T3 or T4

In stage T3, the cancer has spread to tissue adjacent to the prostate or to the seminal vesicles. Stage T4 tumors have spread to organs near the prostate, such as the bladder.

Stage N+ or M+

Cancer has spread to pelvic lymph nodes (N+) or to lymph nodes, organs, or bones distant from the prostate (M+).

Expanded Summary of Staging Systems	Whitmore-Jewett System	TNN System
In the earliest stage, prostate cancer can't be felt during a DRE. It is said to be found "incidentally" during BPH surgery. Biopsied tissue at this stage is less than 5 percent cancerous. Because it is confined to the prostate, small, and low-grade, some doctors recommend "watchful waiting" rather than curative treatment.	A1	T1a
The cancer is not *palpable* (it can't be felt during a DRE) and is found incidentally, during BPH surgery. More than 5 percent of the biopsied tissue is cancerous.	A2	T1b
The cancer is not palpable, but the PSA is elevated and cancer may be found in samples from a needle biopsy.	A3	T1c
Cancer is felt during DRE but is a small nodule confined to less than half of one side of the prostate.	B1N	T2a
Cancer is palpable during DRE and is found in more than half of one side. B1 T2b Cancer is palpable during DRE and is found in both lobes, but there's no evidence that it has spread beyond the prostate.	B2	T2c
Cancer occupies one side and is growing outside the capsule.	C1	T3a
Cancer is in both sides and is growing outside the prostate.	C1	T3c
Cancer has spread to the seminal vesicles.	C2	T3c

Cancer has spread to the bladder neck, rectum, or external sphincter, or all three.	C2	T4a
Cancer has spread to other areas in the pelvis.	C2	T4b
There is no cancer found in the lymph nodes.	—	N0
2 cm or a smaller amount of cancer has spread to lymph nodes.	D1	N1 (N+)
2 to 5 cm of cancer has spread to lymph nodes.	D1	N2 (N+)
5 cm or a greater amount of cancer has spread to lymph nodes.	D1	N3 (N+)
Cancer has not spread beyond pelvic tissues and lymph nodes.	—	M0
Cancer has metastasized beyond the pelvis to bones and perhaps other areas.	D2	M1 (M+)

Resources

American Cancer Society
15999 Clifton Road NE
Atlanta, GA 30329-4251
Phone: (800) 227-2345
www.cancer.org

American Urological Association
1000 Corporate Boulevard
Linthicum, MD 21090
Phone: (800) 828-7866
www.urologyhealth.org

Cancer Care, Inc.
275 Seventh Avenue
New York, NY 10001
Phone: (800) 813-HOPE
www.cancercare.org

National Cancer Institute
NCI Office of Communications and Education
Public Inquiries Office
6116 Executive Boulevard, Suite 300
Bethesda, MD 20892
Phone: (800) 422-6237)
www.nci.nih.gov

National Coalition for Cancer Survivorship

1010 Wayne Avenue, Suite 770
Silver Spring, MD 20910
Phone: (888) 650-9127
www.canceradvocacy.org

National Comprehensive Cancer Network

275 Commerce Drive, Suite 300
Fort Washington, PA 19034
Phone: (215) 690-0300
ww.nccn.com

The New Prostate Cancer InfoLink

P.O. Box 66355
Virginia Beach, VA 23466,
http://prostatecancerinfolink.net/

Patient Advocates for Advance Cancer Treatments (PAACT)

P.O. Box 141695
Grand Rapids, MI 49514
Phone: (616) 453-1477
www.paactusa.org

Prostate Cancer Foundation

1250 Fourth Street
Santa Monica, CA 90401
Phone: (800) 757-2873
www.pcf.org

The Prostate Net, Inc.
P.O. Box 2192
Secaucus, NJ 07096
Phone: (888) 477-6763
www.ProstateNet.org

Us Too!
5003 Fairview Avenue
Downers Grove, IL 60515
Phone: (630) 795-1002
Toll free: (800) 808-7866
www.ustoo.org

ZERO—The Project to End Prostate Cancer
10 G Street, NE, Suite 601
Washington, DC 20002
Phone: (202) 463-9455
www.zerocancer.org

Glossary

A

acute bacterial prostatitis: a sudden severe prostate infection caused by bacteria.

adjuvant therapy: a treatment added to the primary treatment.

adrenal glands: a pair of small glands, one on top of each kidney, that produce small amounts of the male hormone testosterone.

agonist: a drug that simulates physiologic activity at cell receptors stimulated by naturally occurring substances.

alpha-adrenergic agonists: vasoconstrictors (substances that constrict the blood vessels); decongestants.

anastomosis: surgical reattachment of the urethra to the bladder neck after prostatectomy.

androgen blockade: therapy used to eliminate male sex hormones in the body.

androgen deprivation: a treatment that prevents male hormones, principally testosterone, from feeding prostate cancer cells.

androgen-independent cancer: a prostate malignancy that does not depend on male hormones to grow and divide.
androgens: male hormones, including testosterone.

anemia: low red blood cell count.

angiogenesis: the growth of blood vessels.

antagonist: in medicine, a substance that blocks the action of a drug, hormone, or cell.

antiandrogen: a substance that saturates androgen receptors in the prostate and blocks access of testosterone and DHT to those receptors.

anticholinergic agents: drugs that block the neurotransmitter acetylcholine. May be used for urinary urgency.

antibody: substances the body produces to defend against disease.

antioxidants: chemicals (including nutrients such as vitamins A, C, and E) that reduce or prevent oxidation, especially within tissues.

apoptosis: the normal cell death and replacement process.

atypia: variation (indicating disease) in the appearance of the centers of body cells as viewed under a microscope. *See also* prostatic intraepithelial neuroplasia (PIN).

autologous donation: giving your own blood to be used if you need a transfusion during or after surgery.

B

B-mode acquisition and targeting (BAT): an ultrasound positioning system used in the radiation treatment of prostate cancer to localize targets that may move from one treatment day to the next.

benign: in medicine, noncancerous.

benign prostatic hyperplasia (BPH): prostate enlargement caused by growth of tissue surrounding the urethra.

beta carotene: a nutrient related to vitamin A that is found in dark green and dark yellow fruits and vegetables.

biomarkers: naturally occurring body substances whose fluctuations sometimes indicate cancer.

biopsy: removal of a sample of body tissue for pathological examination.

bisphosphonates: a class of drugs used to prevent or treat osteoporosis.

bone marrow: the soft, spongy centers of large bones where blood cells are made.

bone scan: an imaging study that creates images of bones on a computer screen for diagnosis.

brachytherapy: a procedure in which radioactive seeds are implanted in the body to kill cancer cells.

C

cancer: disease characterized by uncontrolled growth and spread of abnormal cells.

castration level: little or no measurable PSA, as would be achieved by surgical castration.

CAT scan: computerized axial tomography. *See* computerized tomography scan.

central zone: refers to the prostate gland's muscular central zone, which prevents semen from backing up into the bladder during ejaculation.

chemical castration: the use of drugs to reduce testosterone to the level that would be achieved with orchiectomy.

chemotherapy: treatment with anticancer drugs.

chronic bacterial prostatitis: persistent and recurrent inflammation of the prostate caused by bacteria.

Cialis: a PDE-5 inhibitor used to treat impotence and erectile dysfunction; generic, tadalafil.

clinical stage: the suspected extent of cancer's spread using evidence gathered from pretreatment testing. *See* pathologic stage; stage.

colony stimulating factors: drugs that promote white blood cell production.

colostomy: a surgical procedure in which the large intestine is routed to an opening in the body through which fecal waste passes to an external bag.

computerized tomography scan (CT or CAT scan): a diagnostic method that uses computerized X-ray images to create a three-dimensional picture of an internal part of the body.

conformal EBRT: a type of external beam radiation therapy in which the radiation beams are more precisely targeted at a patient's tumor than is the case in conventional EBRT.

continence: in medicine, voluntary control over urination and defecation.

corpora cavernosa: the two parallel chambers of the penis that fill with blood to produce an erection.

corpus spongiosum: a central chamber in the penis through which the urethra passes.

cryoablation: destruction of diseased or damaged tissue by freezing.

cryolumpectomy: a procedure in which supercooled cryo-probes are used to destroy a tumor and a minimal amount of surrounding tissue rather than the entire gland in which the tumor resides.

cryoprobes: supercooled instruments used in cryotherapy.

cryosurgery: *see* cryoablation.

cryotherapy: a medical treatment that destroys abnormal tissues by freezing.

CT scan: see computerized tomography scan.

D

debulking: in oncology, reducing the size of a tumor with one treatment, such as hormone therapy or chemotherapy, to facilitate another treatment, such as radiation, cryoablation, or surgery.

deep venous thrombosis: blood clots in the deep veins of the legs.

DEH: *see* diethylstilbestrol.

Denonvillier's fascia: a thin sheet of tissue that separates the prostate and the rectum.

DHT: *see* dihydrotestosterone.

diethylstilbestrol (DES): a form of estrogen.

differentiated: in pathology, a term applied to cells with distinct borders and centers.

diffuse: widespread, scattered, or dispersed.

digital rectal examination (DRE): a diagnostic procedure in which a doctor inserts a gloved, lubricated finger into a man's rectum and feels through the back rectal wall for abnormalities.

dihydrotestosterone (DHT): a potent male hormone to which testosterone is converted in the prostate.

DRE: *see* digital rectal examination.

E

EBRT: *see* external beam radiation therapy.

ejaculatory duct: a channel leading from the seminal vesicle and the vas deferens through the prostate that carries semen out of the body at the time of ejaculation.

endoscope: a long, slender medical instrument equipped with a small camera for examining the interior of an organ or performing surgery.

epididymis: a thin, tightly coiled tube that carries sperm from the testicle to the vas deferens.

epidural: the space between the wall of the spinal canal and the covering of the spinal cord; an anesthetic injection or infusion into this space.

estrogen: a sex hormone that regulates women's reproduction, sometimes used as hormone therapy to treat prostate cancer in men.

external beam radiation therapy (EBRT; XRT): a procedure that uses radiation to destroy cancer from outside the body.

extravasation injury: damage that occurs around the injection site when chemotherapy drugs leak into nearby tissues.

F

Foley catheter: an indwelling catheter—a tube usually inserted for the removal of body waste—the remains in the urethra and bladder until removed.

follicle-stimulating hormone (FSH): a substance that stimulates the testicles to produce testosterone.

free PSA: protein specific antigens that circulate in the blood and are not attached to protein molecules.

free radicals: oxidants; unstable high-energy particles in the body that damage cells.

G

Gleason score: a number between 2 and 10 in a system of grading prostate cancer cells. The lower the number, the closer to normal the cells appear. In general, the higher the number, the more aggressive the tumor.

grade: in oncology, a measure of tumor cells' abnormality and aggressiveness.

granulocytopenia: low white blood cell count.

gynecomastia: breast enlargement and tenderness in men.

H

hematospermia: blood in the semen.

hematuria: blood in the urine.

high-dose-rate implantation (HDR): a brachytherapy procedure in which very high-energy radioactive wires are implanted, left in the body for a short time, then removed.

hormone therapy: in prostate cancer, a treatment whose purpose is to block the body's production, circulation, or absorption of testosterone.

hyperplasia: a benign growth, a thickening or overgrowth of cells.

I

immobilization device: a form-fitting apparatus that helps patients lie perfectly still during external beam radiation therapy.

impotence: the inability to have an erection.

IMRT: *see* intensity-modulated radiation therapy.

incontinence: *see* urinary incontinence.

infusion: in medicine, a method of introducing ("dripping") fluids, including drugs, into the bloodstream.

intensity-modulated radiation therapy (IMRT): in external beam radiation therapy, a technique using multiple small beams that come together to form a single conformal radiation beam.

K

Kegel exercises: a type of muscle training that involves systematically tightening and releasing the urinary sphincter to control the flow of urine.

L

laparoscope: an endoscope (a thin, camera-equipped medical instrument) inserted through a small incision in the abdomen for examination or surgery.

laparoscopic pelvic lymphadenectomy: removal of lymph nodes, using a laparoscope, for pathological examination.

Levitra: a PDE-5 inhibitor used to treat erectile dysfunction or impotence; generic, vardenafil.

LHRH: *see* luteinizing hormone releasing hormone.

LHRH agonist: a substance that tells the pituitary gland to stop producing LHRH.

linear accelerator: a high-energy X-ray treatment machine.

lumpectomy: surgical removal of a tumor and a minimal amount of surrounding tissue rather than the entire gland in which the tumor resides.

luteinizing hormone releasing hormone (LHRH): a substance that stimulates the pituitary gland to release luteinizing hormone.

luteinizing hormone (LH): a substance that stimulates the testicles to produce testosterone.

lycopene: a red pigment (a form of carotenoid) that gives tomatoes their red color and that may help prevent prostate cancer.

lymph: thin clear fluid containing white blood cells that travels through the body's lymphatic system and helps fight infection and disease.

lymphadenectomy: a procedure in which lymph nodes are removed from the body to be examined for cancer.

M

magnetic resonance imaging (MRI): a noninvasive procedure that creates a two-dimensional picture of an internal organ or structure. Magnetic resonance imaging, unlike computerized tomography and X-rays, for example, does not involve radiation.

malignant: in medicine, cancerous.

medical castration: *see* chemical castration.

metastases: cancerous tumors that spread from the original site.

metastasize: spread, as cancer cells.

minilap: *see* minilaparotomy staging pelvic lymphadenectomy.

minilaparotomy staging pelvic lymphadenectomy: a surgical procedure that takes place immediately before retropubic radical prostatectomy. A surgeon removes pelvic lymph nodes through a small incision. If they are found to contain cancer, the prostatectomy is generally canceled.

MRI: *see* magnetic resonance imaging.

multifocal prostate cancer: malignant tumors at several sites within the prostate.

N

nanogram: one billionth of a gram.

needle biopsy: removal of suspected cancer cells through a hollow needle (rather than during a surgical procedure).

neoadjuvant therapy: a treatment given before the primary treatment.

nerve-sparing prostatectomy: surgical removal of the prostate gland that leaves one or both nearby neurovascular bundles intact.

neuropathy: nerve damage expressed as tingling or loss of sensation in the hands or feet.

neurovascular bundles: clusters of nerves near the prostate that enable men to have erections.

neutropenia: low white blood cell count.

nonbacterial prostatitis: inflammation of the prostate from an unknown cause.

O

orchiectomy: surgical castration (removal of the testicles).

organ-confined: of cancer, a tumor or tumors that have not breached the original site.

osteoporosis: a condition of decreased bone mass. This leads to fragile bones which are at an increased risk for fractures.

overflow incontinence: urine leakage that occurs when normal urine flow is blocked and the bladder is always full.

oxidants: *see* free radicals.

P

palliative: used to relieve symptoms rather than cure the underlying illness.

Partin Tables: a tool that uses PSA, clinical stage, and Gleason score to predict how a prostate cancer is likely to behave.

pathologic stage: the actual extent to which a cancer has spread as determined by pathological examination of tissue removed during surgery. *See* clinical stage; stage.

pathologist: a medical doctor who specializes in examinating tissue to make a diagnosis.

patient-controlled analgesia (PCA pump): a pump system for self-administering pain medication. Though patients control their own dosages, the system has safeguards against dosing too much or too often.

PCA pump: *see* patient-controlled analgesia.

PDE-5 inhibitors: drugs used to treat erectile dysfunction and impotence.

pelvic-floor exercises: *see* Kegel exercises.

percutaneous: through unbroken skin.

perineum: the area between the anus and the scrotum.

peripheral zone: the largest part of the prostate, containing about three-fourths of the glands in the prostate.

permanent seed implant (PSI): the permanent implantation of radioactive seeds in the prostate gland.

PET scan: *see* positron emission tomography scan.

phytoestrogens: naturally occurring estrogen-like compounds found in plants.

PIN: *see* prostatic intraepithelial neoplasia.

pituitary gland: located at the base of the brain, the master gland of the endocrine system.

planning study: preparations made for the delivery of radiation therapy.

pneumatic stockings: devices worn on the legs during and after surgery to improve circulation by repeatedly inflating and deflating.

positive margin: cancer identified at the cut surface (insision) of the prostate after surgical removal.

positron emission tomography (PET) scan: a computerized image of body tissues' metabolic activity to determine the presence of disease.

prostate gland: a firm partly muscular chestnut sized gland in males at the base of the bladder; produces a secretion that is the fluid part of semen.

ProstaScint: a staging tool similar to a bone scan except that it finds "hot spots" in soft tissue rather than bones.

prostate capsule: the membrane that encases the numerous small glands of the prostate.

prostate-specific antigen (PSA): a protein manufactured by the prostate to help liquefy semen. Elevated PSA levels can signal prostate disease.

prostatic intraepithelial neoplasia (PIN): cell abnormalities sometimes described as precancerous. *See also* atypia.

prostatitis: inflammation of the prostate.

PSA: *see* prostate-specific antigen.

PSA velocity: the rate at which PSA levels rise.

pubis: one of the pelvic bones.

pulmonary embolism: a blood clot in the lung.

R

radiation oncologist: a medical doctor who specializes in using radiation to treat cancer.

radical laparoscopic prostatectomy: surgical removal of the prostate through a small abdominal incision using an endoscope.

radical perineal prostatectomy: a surgical procedure in which the prostate is removed through an incision in the perineum.

radical prostatectomy: surgical removal of the prostate, seminal vesicles, and pelvic lymph nodes.

radical retropubic prostatectomy: a surgical procedure in which the prostate seminal vesicles, and pelvic lymph nodes are removed through an incision in the lower abdomen.

radioactive seeds: energy-emitting pellets implanted to kill cancer cells.

radioresistant: of tumors, those that are not easily destroyed by radiation therapy.

S

salvage therapy: in prostate cancer, a follow-up treatment used when the primary treatment has failed to eradicate the disease.

saturation biopsy: a biopsy in which specimens are obtained at 5mm intervals throughout the prostate. Carried out through the perineum under ultrasound guidance.

seed implantation: a procedure in which radioactive seeds are placed in the body to kill cancer cells.

semen: a milky liquid produced by the seminal vesicles to carry sperm out of the body.

seminal fluid: Fluid from the prostate and other sex glands that help transport sperm during orgasm.

seminal vesicles: small organs alongside the prostate that manufacture semen.

sepsis: a serious illness caused by severe infection of the bloodstream by a toxin-producing bacteria, virus, or fungus.

stage: of cancer, the extent to which a tumor has spread from its primary site. See clinical stage; pathologic stage.

staging pelvic lymphadenectomy: removal of pelvic lymph nodes to determine whether cancer has spread from the prostate.

stress urinary incontinence: involuntary leakage of urine caused by activity or the sudden movement involved in sneezing, coughing, or laughing.

surgical castration: see orchiectomy.

T

3D global mapping biopsy: *see* saturation biopsy.

temporary seed implant: *see* high-dose-rate implantation (HDR).

testes: *see* testicles.

testicles: the principal organs where the male hormone testosterone is produced.

testosterone: the predominant male hormone, responsible for most male-related traits.

thrombocytopenia: low blood platelet level.

TNM staging system: method of classifying malignant tumors with respect to primary tumor, involvement of regional lymph nodes, and presence or absence of metastastes.

transrectal ultrasound (TRUS): an imaging technique in which sound waves produce a "picture" of the prostate and abnormalities it might contain.

transurethral resection of the prostate (TURP): surgery to remove prostate tissue through the urethra to treat benign prostatic hyperplasia.

TRUS: *see* transrectal ultrasound.

tumor: a mass of abnormal cells, which may be malignant (cancerous) or benign (noncancerous).

tumor markers: *see* biomarkers.

TURP: see transurethral resection of the prostate.

U

unifocal prostate cancer: a single malignant tumor within the prostate.

ureters: tubes that carry urine from the kidneys to the bladder.

urethra: the duct through which urine leaves the body; also, in males, the genital duct.

urethral stricture: narrowing of the urethra caused by scar tissue that forms after surgery.

urethrorectal fistula: a hole between the digestive and urinary tracts.

urge incontinence: the inability to hold urine long enough to reach a restroom.

urinary bladder: the organ in which urine is stored after leaving the kidneys and before leaving the body.

urinary incontinence: inability to control the leaking of urine from the body.

urinary sphincter: the ring of muscle that contracts to prevent urine from leaking.

urologist: a physician who has special knowledge of the male and female urinary tract and the male reproductive organs.

V

vas deferens: singular form of vasa deferentia.
vasa deferentia: the tubes that carry sperm out of the testicles.

vasodilator: a drug that widens blood vessels.

venous access device: a port, under the skin, usually in the chest area, for accessing veins to administer medications intravenously.

Viagra: a PDE-5 inhibitor used to treat erectile dysfunction or impotence; generic, sildenafil citrate.

W

Whitmore-Jewett staging system: a method of describing prostate cancer's spread, less commonly used than the TNM staging system.

X

XRT: *see* external beam radiation therapy.

Index

B

benign prostatic hyperplasia (BPH), 2, 12, 13, 17, 19, 36
  symptoms, 13
  treatment options, 13
benign tumor, 6
beta-carotene, 12
Bicalutamide, 75
biofeedback, 107, 118
biomarkers, 18, 19
biopsy, 18, 19, 25, 34
  complications, 24
  preparing for, 23
  risk factors, 24
  side effects, 24
bisphosphonates, 79, 83, 84
bladder, 13, 39, 43, 68
  control issues, 105
  damage from radiation, 60
  obstruction, 75
  spasms, 46
bladder surgery, 19
bleeding, 24, 74
blood clot, 23, 37, 41, 49, 70, 113
  impaired, 96
blood tests, 56
blood thinners, 23, 37, 49, 56
blood transfusions, 38, 91, 118
blood vessels, 6, 68, 73, 110
bloodless field, 38
blue haze, 112
B-mode acquisition and targeting (BAT), 62
bone health, 83
bone loss, 78, 79
bone marrow, 95, 118

bone metastases, 71, 79, 83
  treatment options, 83
bone pain, 69, 75, 81, 86
  reduction, 87
bone scan, 27
bowel injury, 49, 54
bowel movements, pain during, 66
bowel regularity, 45
brachytherapy, 53, 64, 67
  preparing for, 54, 55
  recovery, 58
brain fog, 99
breast cancer, 9
breast enlargement, 76
breast tenderness, 74, 76

C

cabazitaxel, 86, 89
cancer, 6
  cells, 25, 26
  clinical stage, 25
  Gleason score, 26
  grading, 22, 24, 25, 39
  pathologic stage, 25
  recurrence, 47, 116
  staging systems, 25
candidates for
  chemotherapy, 88
  hormonal therapy, 78
  radiation therapy, 51, 59
  surgery, 30
carboplatin, 89
cardiologist, 112
cardiovascular risks, 77
Casodex, 75
castration level, 73, 75, 76
catheterization, 19, 50

prostatic uretha, 39
prostatitis, 12, 13, 17, 19
  acute bacterial, 14
  symptoms, 13
proteins, 84
proton and neutron beam
  therapy technologies, 62
Provenge, 81
PSA blood test, 16, 18, 47, 59,
  63, 116
PSA levels, 19–20, 78
  bump, 67
  elevation, 67, 81, 84, 116
  guidelines, 20
PSA velocity (PSAV), 20
pseudoephedrine, 106
pulmonary embolism, 42

Q

Quadramet, 84

R

race and ethnicity as risk factor, 9
radiation oncologist, 52, 54
radiation therapy, 47, 51–70,
  71, 105
  candidates for, 64
  complications, 65–67
  hormone treatment, 53
  risk factors, 65–67
  and salvage therapy, 68
  short-term   complications,
  66
  side effects, 65–67
  spot radiation, 69
  types, 52, 53, 67
radical laparoscopic prostatectomy, 34

radical retropubic prostatectomy, 31, 32, 38, 51, 68,
  71, 105
radioactive isotope, 69
radioactive seeds, 53, 54, 57
  expelled, 67
radioisotopes, 84
radiopharmaceuticals, 84
Radium-223, 84
rectal blood, 48
rectal mucus, 48
rectum, 2, 4, 18, 21, 56, 57, 59,
  68, 108
  damage from radiation, 60,
  66
recurrence, 64, 65, 116
red blood cell production, 91
relaxation techniques, 118
reproductive system, 90
retropubic incision, 33
ringing in ears, 98, 99
risk factors, for prostate cancer, 8–11
robotic laparoscopic prostatectomy, 35
  advantages, 36
  disadvantages, 36

S

salvage prostatectomy, 117
salvage therapy, 68, 69, 116,
  117
Samarium-153, 84
saturation biopsy, 22
scrotum, 4, 73, 74, 108, 114
secondary hormone manipu-
  lations, 80, 81, 82
seed implantation, 53, 55, 69.

About the Author

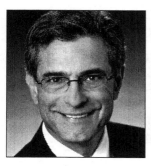

Arthur S. Centeno, M.D., is a board-certified urologist in private practice at Urology San Antonio in San Antonio, Texas. He treats prostate cancer patients through surgery, brachytherapy, and cryo-surgery.

"I decided I wanted to be a doctor when I was twelve years old and while visiting my grandfather in the hospital and I realized I wanted to help people. My philosophy of medicine has evolved over the years. I have learned it is important that doctors be more than medical technologists—they must also be empathetic to patients and families. This became so clear to me when my wife died of breast cancer in 2001. I teach my medical students that we are dealing with people, not just diseases."

Dr. Centeno is a graduate of the University of Texas Health Science Center in San Antonio, Texas. He completed his surgical internship and residency in urology at the University of Texas Medical Branch in Galveston, Texas, and earned a Master of Medical

Sciences degree at that institution's Graduate School of Biomedical Sciences.

Dr. Centeno is a member of the American Urological Association and Sigma Xi Scientific Research Society, and is a Fellow of the American College of Surgeons. He has two children, Rebecca and Everett.

Dr. Centeno may be reached at www.urology-sanantonio.com.

Consumer Health Titles from Addicus Books

Visit our online catalog at www.AddicusBooks.com

To Order Books:
Visit us online at: www.AddicusBooks.com
Call toll free: (800) 888-4741

For discounts on bulk purchases, call our Special Sales
Department at (402) 330-7493.
Or email us at: info@Addicus Books.com

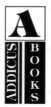

Addicus Books
P. O. Box 45327
Omaha, NE 68145

*Addicus Books is dedicated to publishing consumer health books
that comfort and educate.*